The Practitioner
as Teacher

Cartoons by Martin Davies
Illustrations by Chartwell Illustrators

For Baillière Tindall
Senior Commissioning Editor: Jacqueline Curthoys
Project Editor: Karen Gilmour

The Practitioner as Teacher

Edited by

Sue Hinchliff MSc BA RGN RNT

Head of Continuing Professional Development,
Royal College of Nursing Institute,
Royal College of Nursing of the United Kingdom,
London

SECOND EDITION

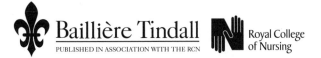

Baillière Tindall
PUBLISHED IN ASSOCIATION WITH THE RCN

Royal College
of Nursing

EDINBURGH LONDON NEW YORK PHILADELPHIA SYDNEY TORONTO 1999

BAILLIÈRE TINDALL
An imprint of Harcourt Brace and Company Limited

© Harcourt Brace and Company Limited 1999

First published 1992 by Scutari Press
Reprinted by Baillière Tindall and copyright transfered 1996
Second edition 1999

ISBN 0 702 024473

British Library Cataloguing in Publication Data
A catalogue record for this book is available from the British Library.

Library of Congress Cataloging in Publication Data
A catalog record for this book is available from the Library of Congress.

Note
Medical knowledge is constantly changing. As new information becomes
available, changes in treatment, procedures, equipment and the use of drugs
become necessary. The editors, contributors and the publishers have, as far as
it is possible, taken care to ensure that the information given in this text is
accurate and up to date. However, readers are strongly advised to confirm
that the information, especially with regard to drug usage, complies with
latest legislation and standards of practice.

Publisher's Note
In this edition we have alternated the use of 'he' and 'she' for students
with each new chapter (the gender of teachers, patients and relatives
vary throughout). This is the publisher's usual style and not that of the RCN.

The
publisher's
policy is to use
**paper manufactured
from sustainable forests**

Printed in China
NPCC/01

Contents

Reflective learning; Feedback; The learning environment; The status of assessors; Conclusion; Glossary; References; Further reading

List of contributors

Anne Eaton BSc RCNTCertEd RNT RM RGN
Education/VQ Adviser, Royal College of Nursing of the United Kingdom,
London, UK

Sue Howard MA DNT DNCert RHV RGN
Education Adviser, Royal College of Nursing of the United Kingdom,
London, UK

Sally Thomson, MA(Ed) BEd(Hons) DipNEd RGN RMN
Assistant Director – Education, Department of Nursing Policy and Practice,
Royal College of Nursing of the United Kingdom, London, UK

Preface
to the second edition

Nurses have always been educators, and from the time of Florence Nightingale this has been an expressed component of the role. They have not, however, always been formally prepared to teach. It was during the 1970s that nurses were first offered any preparation for their teaching role, and this has continued to this day as some form of teaching and assessing course, related to the practice area and validated through one of the National Boards. The length and level of the courses may vary, but each sets out to provide some basic instruction in how to set about teaching either nurses, patients/clients, other health care professionals or support workers.

The first edition of this text was published in 1992 to meet the needs of practitioners at that time, whether or not they had received any help with preparation for teaching. Nursing, however, and nurse education with it, has moved on in the past few years. The initial preparation for practice has evolved over this period; the setting in which it occurs has changed, with the move of pre and postregistration education into the world of higher education and the continuing shift in practice towards the community; the way in which education is commissioned and delivered has altered; and, significantly, those with whom we work to deliver care have changed during this time, with fewer registered nurses and a greater number of support workers, trained to National Vocational Qualification standards.

For these reasons, it seemed timely, with the second edition of this book, to change radically the way in which this text is structured. A new team of writers was commissioned, all with an expert education brief within the Royal College of Nursing. As a team, we worked closely together to identify the sort of information a practitioner would need if he or she were to feel confident and competent to teach in today's health care workplace. We think that we have achieved this.

We have produced a second edition that addresses the context in which our practice and the preparation for it is set. We have explored some of the theories that underpin the ways in which learning takes place. We have unpicked the process of learning and teaching, and explored the component parts. Above all, we have tried to help you to see the ways in which you can help someone – a patient or relative, a student nurse or medical student, a health care assistant – learn what you have to teach them.

In doing all this, we have attempted to retain the practical emphasis of the first edition, using activities to cause you to think, apply, find out and be active in your learning rather than just a passive recipient. It is very much a book that sets out to help you to 'know how' rather than just 'know what'.

We hope we will be of use to you and accompany you on a wealth of learning and teaching journeys, and that you will enjoy helping others to learn—with confidence on both sides.

1998   Sue Hinchliff

Preface

to the first edition

The impetus for this book came from two points. The first arose from my current post as Course Director for the Diploma in Professional Studies in Nursing by distance learning. On this course the students study a pair of units entitled *The Reflective Practitioner*, during which they are presented with material on a variety of themes relating to reflective practice, such as coping with stress, improving communication skills, becoming more competent at reflecting on what they do as they do it as well as after it's done, becoming professionally more assertive, improving decision-making abilities and so on.

While we were planning the curriculum for these units it became clear that we should be offering the students a learning package on how to develop their skills in teaching their colleagues, patients, clients and relatives and furthermore, how to reflect on these developing competencies in order to build on them. And so the idea for a distance learning package on *The Practitioner as Teacher* was born.

Since all the chapters have been written by different authors, you may perceive some differences in style and approach. I have made no attempt to edit these variations out. The whole tone of the book is that of a teacher talking you through the topics being discussed, and as all teachers have different teaching styles, I felt that you should be exposed here to such variety. You will notice that the book is written in the first person, that is, in a personal tone, rather than in the more formal style that you are used to in academic texts.

I was concerned that the book adopt an interactive format, where readers are urged to reflect on what they are reading, question their practice, examine the theory behind interventions, try out new approaches, etc. In fact, I saw the emerging package not so much as a book but more as a workbook, a resource to be actively *used* rather than just *read* and not just used once, but referred to many times throughout practice.

It is for this reason that you will notice that we have included quite a lot of 'white space', that is, space within the text for you to add your own notes as you read. I am aware that some of you will see it as verging on the sacrilegious to write on a book, but I am encouraging you to do just that here! Use it to jot down your responses to the activities that we provide. It will be useful to be able to refer back to them later. This book should end up as a very personal document, which records your progress in becoming a competent teacher.

Please don't try to save time by skipping the activities. Each one has been designed to make a point that will be learned more effectively by completing the activity. You will note that each one is followed by a comment, but that there are no right or wrong answers, just as there is no one right way to teach a topic, but lots of individual approaches.

With regards to the structure of the book, since all readers will be familiar with the nursing process, I decided to use that systematic approach here. The chapters are of equal importance, even though they are not of equal length. The book opens with a chapter on the nature of teaching and learning, to set the scene. It continue with four chapters which focus on

- assessing learning needs
- planning for teaching
- the process of teaching
- evaluating teaching and learning

It concludes with a chapter which draws the threads of the preceding material together, in applying the contents to the practice setting.

Suggestions for further reading are included at the end of each chapter, annotated to indicate their usefulness and what the reader might hope to get out of them. At the end of the text you will find a composite glossary of words with which some readers may be unfamiliar. To indicate that a word appears in the Glossary, it is printed in bold where it first appears in the text.

We wanted the book to be equally useful, whatever the clinical speciality of the reader, whether a midwife, a nurse caring for old people, or a community psychiatric nurse and to be relevant at any stage of practice. I hope it will be used during courses leading to registration, for I have long felt that we leave learners somewhat in the lurch when it comes to teaching. They may know *what* to teach but strategies for getting the message across effectively are often not imparted until towards the end of, or after training, by which time many opportunities may have been lost.

A note about terminology

We have tended to use the term **teacher-practitioner** throughout, to denote the person who is doing the teaching. This term was chosen to indicate that the teacher is primarily a practitioner rather than a trained teacher. For the person who is being taught, we have most commonly used the word **student**, whether that person is, in fact, a student of nursing or midwifery, or is a patient, client or relative.

We have tried to avoid the use of gender-specific language, without resorting too frequently to cumbersome combinations of his/her, etc. Where the masculine or feminine pronoun has been used, this should not be taken to imply that a person of that gender is the usual occupant of the position referred to.

Whoever uses this book, in whatever circumstances, I hope that you will gain enjoyment and expertise from doing so. Above all, I hope that it will serve to open the door for you to some of the excitement, challenges and satisfaction that teaching has to offer. In both teaching and learning there's a lot of fun to be had, once you become confident enough to let yourself experience it. This book is designed to give you that confidence.

Sue Hinchliff

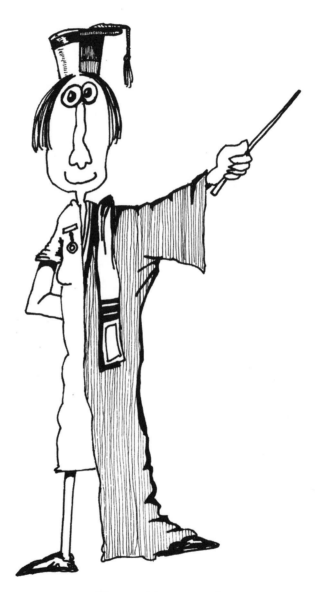

The practitioner as teacher

1 The nature of teaching and learning

Sally Thomson

INTRODUCTION

Regardless of whether you practise as a nurse, midwife or health visitor, in a GP practice, community or hospital setting, teaching is an important aspect of your role, and you have little choice about whether or not you continue to learn.

As teaching and learning are so intertwined, you, as someone who teaches about nursing, may choose to link some of your learning objectives into your performance review so that you are able to maximise upon opportunities. Teaching and learning for yourself and others can be streamlined, to the advantage of both you as a learner and a teacher, and also those who will learn from you and who, vicariously, may also teach you.

Your 'student' may be training for one of the registers, be a patient or client, a relative, a colleague undergoing an orientation programme, a new doctor in the team or a member of the ancillary staff. Regardless of who the student is, she is entitled to the best possible standard of teaching that you can offer. You may be learning simply for pleasure, as a purposeful activity to be able to re-register, as part of your own professional development, or to study towards a formal academic award. As you gain experience and insight into this crucial aspect of your work, the complex relationship between teaching and learning will become apparent, as the two roles – student and teacher – merge, each learning from, and facilitating learning in, the other.

Teaching is a behaviour open to wide interpretation; it is something that can be learned about, developed and refined by improving your knowledge base,

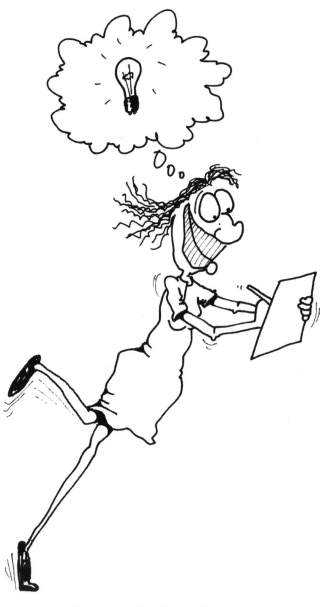

The nature of teaching and learning

practising and reflecting on your practice. This chapter sets out to help you to develop a personal working definition of teaching and considers the qualities of both effective and ineffective teaching, as a basis for analysing ways of developing your teaching style.

Teaching cannot be considered in isolation from how people learn. We will link different teaching theories to models that will help to structure your teaching and develop your own ways of learning. A brief consideration of the factors that affect learning will allow you to maximise every teaching and learning opportunity that you have. Teaching also occurs through the processing of experience with another, and to explore this idea, supervision, mentorship and preceptorship are briefly explored as the foundation for the rest of the book.

Lifelong learning and evidence-based practice are two major themes that are present in all chapters of this book, and, as a beginning, the two are introduced in this chapter.

Finally, a framework for integrating all the ideas is suggested as a way of structuring the teaching programme in your practice setting.

The words that appear in bold type throughout this chapter are explained in the glossary, which can be found at the end of the chapter.

LEARNING OBJECTIVES

After reading this chapter, you should be able to:

- identify your pathway towards lifelong learning
- explain the differences between mentorship, supervision and preceptorship
- discuss the significance of evidence-based practice
- evaluate your teaching style and set objectives for developing this
- consider factors influencing learning and use these yourself and with your students
- describe and utilise four families of teaching that underpin a curriculum (don't worry if you don't understand this one yet!)

FOUNDATION THEMES

Lifelong learning

The term 'lifelong learning' is a contemporary expression, linked to the overall notion that if all individuals in society take responsibility for their own development, we will create a 'learning society', as described in the Dearing Report on higher education (National Committee of Inquiry into Higher Education, 1997).

ACTIVITY 1.1

Take a few minutes to consider the term 'lifelong learning' and consider what this means for you in your professional life. You may choose to explore the definition by referring to texts, but your own view is a good starting point.

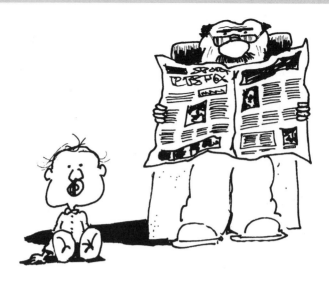

Lifelong learning

Apart from the obvious statement that we are to learn all our lives, you may have thoughts about the constant development of your knowledge and how this will influence your practice, the way in which you think about care and the repertoire of skills that you continually need to develop and update.

Lifelong learning may present itself as opportunities for formal courses that are assessed and carry credit at a given academic level. For example, you may be reading this book as part of your studies for a course at academic level 2 or 3. Equally, it embraces those informal moments when you pursue your learning for yourself or to solve a problem at work. However, learning is an active process and will not happen without you ordering, categorising and evaluating your thoughts.

Lifelong learning may also ensure that you remain flexible and open to change; in fact, it may cause you to initiate developments in care or in your working life. Finally, developing knowledge is a powerful tool, both personally, in terms of growing confidence, and also professionally, as knowledge offers an unshake-able platform for our work. Edwards (1977) begins his challenging read on this issue by quoting Foucalt:

> knowing if one can think differently than one thinks, and perceive
> differently than one sees is absolutely necessary if one is to go on
> looking and reflecting at all. (Foucalt, 1987, p. 8; cited by Edwards,
> 1997)

Lifelong learning provides the philosophy that underpins the requirements for re-registration (UKCC, 1997a). If you are unclear about the requirements for postregistration education and practice (PREP; Box 1.1) this may be a good time to check them out. One thing is certain: you are (or should be) working towards meeting the requirements now. Also, if you have not yet begun to construct your profile, you will need at some point either to begin or to refine your ideas and plans for this. Activity 1.2, although requiring some thought, is extremely worthwhile.

BOX 1.1	*Recommended reading*
	UKCC (1997) *PREP and You.* This short booklet, which the United Kingdom Central Council for Nursing, Midwifery and Health visiting (UKCC) sends to all registered nurses, will explain the requirements in an easily read style.

Before doing Activity 1.2, ensure that you are able to distinguish for yourself the difference between a portfolio and a profile. A portfolio is all the experiences you have had to date. These may be influenced by the sort of person you are, why you chose nursing as a career, significant experiences you have had in nursing and in your personal life, as well as the skills and learning that have taken place since you began nursing. A portfolio might contain contracts, photographs, leaving cards, records of achievement and feedback from performance reviews. A profile is a more focused activity. It may well be that, from your collection of experience in your portfolio, you focus on five or six themes for which you set objectives and which provide the reflective medium for your personal and professional development for the foreseeable future.

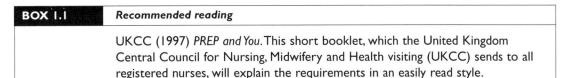

ACTIVITY 1.2

From your portfolio, extract the learning experiences you have had in the past 3 years. You may wish to put these under different headings, for example, courses with an academic credit rating, starting with your preregistration course, then short courses and workshops that you have completed as part of your professional role, then, perhaps to help fulfil your PREP requirements, the learning that you have gained from reflecting on and making sense of experience, and finally, a section for self-generated learning. If you have plans for the future, in terms of either formal study or knowledge and experience that you intend to acquire, it is worth logging this in your profile.

This may be something that you return to develop over a period of time as your experiences increase. This exercise will clearly demonstrate the nature of lifelong learning and the effort you have put into it. If you compare your map of learning with that of a peer, it may help you to identify gaps, either for yourself or to help to meet your client's needs.

This is an important exercise, not only in terms of defining the term 'lifelong learning', but also as a crucial part of your profile and as the foundation of your own professional development plans. You are likely to need to use this record in a variety of ways: as a tool for agreeing learning needs during your performance review, as part of a job application, or if reviewing the skill mix of the nurses in your practice area.

From the initial exploration of lifelong learning, and as you progress through this chapter, you will realise that learning is about change. If you now return to your log of learning experiences and ask the question. 'What changed as a result of the learning?', you will notice that some learning developed client care and some was for your own personal development. Equally, you may note an increase in confidence or new skills in communication that improved your assertiveness.

Evidence-based practice

Consider an everyday aspect of your work, for example, care that you give to clients as a matter of routine. Why do you do it? Are you confident that there is a rationale to support the strategies you are using? Briefly jot down one aspect of care, noting the rationale for its use. Ask your colleagues if they know why this particular strategy is used.

Next time you visit the library, do a quick search to see if you can find literature to support your care and see if there are any conflicting viewpoints. If there are differences of opinion, which option do you think is the best and why? Note this down in your reflective journal. Most importantly, consider why this exercise is so significant.

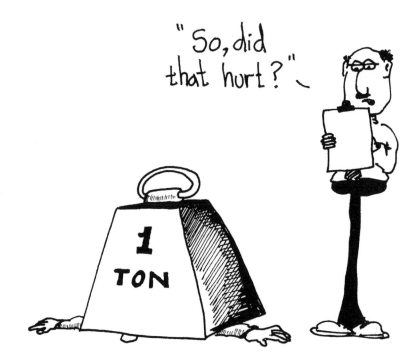

Evidence-based practice

Already, from your reflection, you will know that to practice nursing using evidence requires skills in assessing evidence, analysis, decision-making and reflection. A journal editorial (Editorial, 1998) describes evidence-based nursing as giving quantitative or qualitative meaning to the cause, course, diagnosis, treatment or economics of health problems managed by nurses, and also includes quality assurance and continuing professional development. Evidence-based practice, in effect, bridges the gap that exists between theory and practice by integrating research with practice. This is the first opportunity to perceive the theory – practice gap as an opportunity rather than a weakness.

While it is not practical to debate the nature of research in this chapter, it is evident that knowledge exists in many different forms and emerges from a variety of often opposing research disciplines. Therefore, planning what is best for patients rests on your clinical expertise, patient preferences and research evidence.

THE NATURE OF TEACHING

You may already feel comfortable and reasonably confident in your teaching role or you may be at the other extreme, in beginning to consider how you can develop this aspect of your work. Regardless of where you are in terms of insights into teaching, you may not have thought before about what teaching is. This may be a good point to start.

ACTIVITY 1.4

Think either of yourself when teaching, or a colleague, and note down the behaviour that tells you that teaching is taking place.

You may come up with some conflicting ideas. Also note down any ideals or values that you believe are inherent in the word 'teaching'. Now compare your ideas with the following definitions.

Peters (1977, p. 151) provides a useful starting point for a definition of teaching: 'It includes a host of activities that have in common the structuring of a situation in such a way that something can be learned.'

The use of the word 'structured' suggests a planned, rational approach, so that even if a situation demands that you teach in an impromptu way, you would stop for a couple of minutes, collect your thoughts, assess the resources available to you, think about what your student needs to know and assess her readiness to learn before you begin.

But teaching is not as simple as that. Gage (1978) suggests that, like nursing, it is both an art and a science. The rationality of teaching theories could be viewed, for example, as the scientific approach – using a model of teaching that matches the style of learning – while the art may rest in the use of an analogy to illustrate an idea, or the way in which the teacher relates to the students, sensing when someone is confused in a seemingly intuitive way, or in the use of a particularly imaginative introduction to a topic.

Lawton (1987) portrays the teacher as one 'who enriches the life of a child across a wide range of worthwhile experiences'. We need to substitute 'child' for whoever our student is. It may be useful to consider what a worthwhile experience might be. In professional practice, we have the opportunity to create experiences that can enable students to marry theoretical concepts to the practicalities of reality. A student may have a knowledge of sociology, psychology and physiology, and may be able to write an essay discussing the principles of rehabilitation for a patient who has lost a limb. Think, however, how much more real the student's perception of need might be if she accompanied an occupational therapist on a home visit with the patient before he was discharged; the student would then become more aware of the problem of how to get to a downstairs bathroom in the night, or of the psychological implications of needing two legs to pursue employment, for example, if the patient was a policeman. I doubt that you would disagree that this is a worthwhile experience.

A more difficult consideration may be that of the student nurse on a medical ward placement who asks for a teaching session on orthopaedics when you have no patients within this category on your ward. Is it worthwhile to grant her request? You know that she has an assessment on the subject, but it might be more worthwhile to use the opportunity to discuss a nursing problem that is currently common to several patients in your care and which applies the theoretical knowledge gained from a study day. A difficult dilemma. Lawton, then, may give food for thought.

The notion of what is worthwhile may be further explored by considering the influential work of Rogers (1983, p. 18), who states: 'the primary task of the teacher is to permit the student to learn to feed his or her own curiosity'.

There is a wealth of potential learning in each clinical area that your students can explore if you have the skills to facilitate this and if this is what your students want. Different students may be ready to be curious at differing stages in their course. Capturing the moment when a student knows what she needs to know is important. If, for example, a student is experiencing referrals in practice assessments, can you justify her desire to read about alternative methods of pain control when her drug administration is unsafe? This brings us back again to the debate about what is worthwhile and what you believe the nature of teaching to be.

For an inspiring and enjoyable read, do try Rogers (1983), who describes how a teacher can build on student-centred approaches to teaching, with case study examples. This work is considered a classic and is written in a style that makes it easy to dip into.

Take time now to reflect. Compare the ideas discussed so far with your own thoughts and the notes you made on what teaching is. You may have listed behaviours, such as questioning, that are inherent in the definitions we have discussed. These are, of course, just a few examples from the numerous differing definitions to be found.

You are probably beginning to realise that teaching is rooted in a value system. Your thinking may be in line with mine, or your ideas may be completely unrepresented in the discussion so far; neither of us is wrong. Teaching is a highly personal, and at times, emotional activity. What we all have in common is a marvellous grounding for teaching, from our experience, knowledge, beliefs, ideals and attitudes, and, as our careers progress, from the rich resource of the practice setting in which we each work.

The primary aim of teaching, then, is that in a variety of ways, when it happens, it helps others to learn (Joyce and Weil, 1986).

The place of supervision, mentorship and preceptorship in helping others to learn

It is evident that helping others to learn always rests upon the principles of effective communication; this is addressed later in the chapter. However, these helping relationships are often placed under the umbrella of supervision, mentoring or the role of preceptor. It might be argued that, although the principles of each are the same, there are differences in each role.

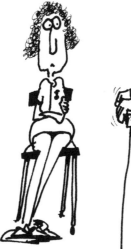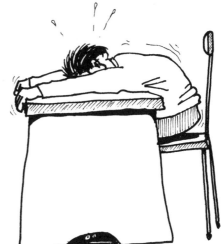

Helping others to learn

ACTIVITY 1.5

Use the guidelines that are issued on the three roles in your place of work and, most importantly, your experience in each role. If you do not have access to these within your own workplace, you may be able to obtain a copy from your local Trust or from a library. Devise a chart to compare and contrast these approaches. If you do not operate in all three roles, ask a colleague to share the work with you. Or it may be something that you develop as a project with those who are facilitated by you. It will certainly have tremendous scope in terms of feedback and the setting of personal objectives.

You will have worked out that differences exist in the process, in the ways of overseeing, in the formality of the exercise, in assessment and evaluation, and in time frames. You may also have discovered that there are many areas of overlap and that many registered nurses get confused about the specifics of each way of working. You may think of displaying your chart where the team with whom you work can see it. It may indicate areas where a small unit seminar may be helpful for the nursing team. Much literature has been written comparing the three roles, and you may wish to underpin your ideas with some reading. The document on standards for preparation of teachers (United Kingdom Central Council for Nursing, Midwifery and Health Visiting, 1997b) has useful definitions of 'mentor' and 'mentorship' as part of their consideration of the lecturer's role. Barton-Wright (1994) develops these ideas to consider how mentoring extends into clinical supervision. Finally, among the wealth of literature on these topics, one to be recommended is the book by Butterworth and Faugier (1992). (The texts are referenced in the further reading section at the end of the chapter.)

CHARACTERISTICS OF AN EFFECTIVE TEACHER

Before reading on, stop to reflect. Think about a teacher whom you would classify as good or even brilliant. Jot down what it was about him or her that was influential. How do your thoughts compare with the points below?

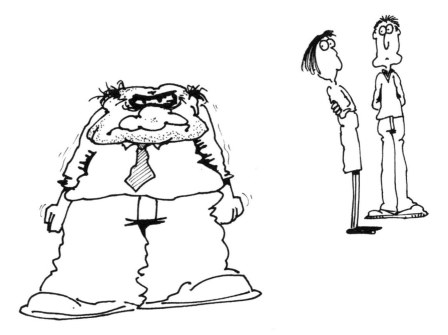

Characteristics of an effective teacher

In general education, the qualities necessary for effective teaching have been widely researched, and you can see from the date of some of the references that ideas do not change over time. Good teaching is promoted by a sound knowledge base (Alulinas, 1978; Fontana, 1972; Henry et al, 1981; Schonell, 1962). Ted Wragg (1984), in a down-to-earth mood, holds that the teacher should know her stuff; Sherman and Blackburn (1974) call for intellectual competence. It is also important for practitioners to be aware of the things they do not know, particularly in caring settings where treatments and practices are changing so rapidly.

The good teacher develops a feeling for the students' emotional needs, social background and cognitive development (Fontana, 1972), and an interest in the welfare of pupils promotes learning (Wragg, 1984). This is particularly pertinent in health care settings, where 'pupils', regardless of who they are, will come from a wide variety of backgrounds, cultures and age groups, so we have to be adaptable to meet such diverse needs. An insight into who and how your student is may help you get the teaching/learning climate right.

Henry (1981) found that the personal background of the teacher affected performance, while Alulinas (1978) discovered the teacher's level of intelligence to be significant. It is not essential to know everything or be very clever, but it helps if you can assess whether the student is able to follow your line of thinking or is completely confused by the variety of interesting facts you offer.

The philosophical stand of the teacher is important (Henry, 1981; Wragg, 1974). Fontana (1972) calls for a unified philosophy of life. The teacher you have referred to may be someone who believes that the relationship with the student is equal, that learning is best achieved by doing something interesting and that students deserve respect.

Peters (1977) refers to the idiosyncrasies of the successful teacher's personality. The profile of characteristics highlighted in the literature is profuse. It includes patience, consideration, emotional stability, maturity and sound judgement (Alulinas, 1978). Wragg (1984) describes an unconventional, experimenting, flexible character; perhaps this is someone who is willing to break from the traditional methods of teaching. Fontana (1972) feels that personal curiosity is important. This may be the teacher who works with the student to discover facts, experiences and relationships between events, rather than telling the student what these are.

Significantly for health professionals, Wragg (1984) found that those teachers who offer minimal criticism and maximise pupil responses are favoured. This is a challenge to one's own practice, since constructive criticism is a vital aspect of the teacher's role. If we do not help students to identify areas in which they have the potential to develop good, as well as correct negative behaviour, we cannot help them to maximise their strengths and minimise their weaknesses. Perhaps we ought to ensure, when giving feedback to students, that we balance the points on which there is a need to improve with the strengths. Additionally, there are times when an unconditional 'That was excellent' without a qualifying 'but' ought to be used. Often, if you ask a student whether she is aware of the areas in which there is a need to improve, she will tell you.

Before we point out the strengths and weaknesses of others, we may wish to demonstrate insight into our own potential and limitations. Fontana (1972) indicates that self-awareness predicts successful teaching and may lead to a confident and assured manner (Sherman and Blackburn 1974) in your teaching style. Not surprisingly, a sense of humour is important, together with a dynamic, pragmatic and approachable air (Schonell 1961). Alulinas (1978) stipulates communication skills, verbal ability and interactive skills, and calls for physical energy and drive.

Discipline, hopefully, is something that we will not have to worry about, except in rare circumstances. However, in our practice, we do need to be aware of the appropriate relationship boundaries. Some of these emerge when considering facilitator style.

Finally, researchers believe that an enduring enthusiasm for teaching (Fontana, 1972; Wragg, 1984), an interest in the subject, and the creation of an effective teaching environment, tend to promote success in teaching and learning encounters (Wragg, 1984; Sheffield, 1974).

From the pupils' perspective, an effective teacher is one who gains credibility from competence, character and intention, is honest and fair, is qualified by experience to know what he or she is talking about and is concerned about the students as well as self. Additionally, the teacher must be 'personalistic', remembering details of the students, as well as being sensitive to their mood and feelings (Burns, 1982).

In nurse education, Howie (1988) describes how role models were chosen in the clinical setting because they were able to communicate effectively and appeared enthusiastic about nursing. Wong (1978) identified nine categories of teacher behaviour considered helpful to student learning (Box 1.2).

BOX 1.2	Wong's (1978) nine categories of helpful teacher behaviour

1. Shows a willingness to answer questions and offer explanations
2. Treats students with interest and respect
3. Uses encouragement and praise
4. Informs students of their progress
5. Uses humour
6. Has a pleasant voice
7. Is accessible to students
8. Supervises effectively
9. Expresses confidence both in self and the student

Marson (1982) collected 49 statements about the characteristics of trained nurses considered to be good at teaching. These covered five areas:

- professional qualities
- managerial abilities
- personality traits
- empathetic qualities
- teaching abilities.

The report is interesting reading, and although written in 1982, the work is still influential and worth reading.

A study of perceptions of best and worst clinical teachers in a faculty of a Canadian university (Morgan and Knox, 1987) revealed that the best clinical teachers were perceived by faculty and students as good role models who enjoyed nursing and teaching and who were skilled and confident in both activities. They were approachable, promoting 'mutual respect'. Students perceived the best teachers to be enthusiastic, non-belittling and encouraging independence. The faculty valued breadth of nursing knowledge, clear explanation and the ability to increase students' interests as important features.

BOX 1.3	Combs's (1965) eight features of an effective teacher

The effective teacher
1. will have an internal (from within the self, i.e. ideas and values) rather than external (e.g. pressure from peers) frame of reference, seeking to understand how things seem to others as a guide for behaviour
2. is more concerned with people and their reactions than with things and events
3. is more concerned with how things seem to people rather than facts
4. seeks to understand the causes of people's behaviour in terms of current thinking, feeling and understanding rather than in terms of forces exerted upon them now or previously
5. trusts others and believes that people have the capacity to solve their own problems
6. sees others as friendly and enhancing rather than hostile or threatening
7. sees others as worthwhile
8. sees people and their behaviour as developing from within rather than as the result of external events; for example, nurses work to give care rather than for financial rewards

Burns (1982) advocates that effective teachers have positive self-concepts, believing that how teachers perceive themselves and students will determine the effectiveness of their teaching. He refers to Combs (1965), who lists eight features of the effective teacher (Box 1.3).

Burns (1982) concludes that how teachers perceive themselves and others will affect their ability to teach.

Are the behaviours that you listed as qualities of a good teacher reflected in any of these research findings? You may find that your definition of teaching in the first activity has crept into your thoughts as you have read this section.

THE INEFFECTIVE TEACHER

As we have seen, the criteria for an effective teacher are wide and varied. It may be useful to consider behaviour that does not facilitate learning, in an attempt to narrow the field. There are valuable lessons to be learned from the following extreme examples.

Student teachers who failed a course of teacher training in general education had difficulties with classroom (for which we might substitute clinical area) management, were unable to relate well to students, displaying poor teaching methods, and had a lack of commitment to the profession (Rickman and Hollowell, 1981).

Alulinas (1978) describes plodding, self-conscious, nervous, easily tired student teachers who were insensitive to learner needs and had a weak impact upon them. Alternatively, the ineffective teacher may be 'big-mouthed', outspoken and disruptive, frequently displaying behaviour that goes against the organisational norm.

Similarly, in the nursing literature, ineffective teaching results when there is a lack of interest from qualified staff, who may distance themselves both physically and psychologically from the students (Marson, 1982). The trained staff may pose a threat when teaching (Wong 1978) so that students are unable to relax sufficiently to enable the kind of dialogue necessary to allow learning. Trained staff may demonstrate a lack of enjoyment of nursing (Morgan and Knox, 1987), be unwilling or unable to answer questions and be insensitive to students' needs (Marson, 1982).

Wong (1978) indicates that staff who act in a superior manner, belittle students, or supervise them too closely, are not successful teachers. Personality clashes may also affect learning (Marson, 1982), although this is not necessarily something that can be avoided. Morgan and Knox (1987) describe poor teachers as being deficient in communication skills.

While in general education a lack of criticism of students is seen as a feature of poor teaching, in professional nursing literature, unsuccessful teachers tend only to emphasise the students' mistakes and weaknesses, correcting these in the presence of others (Wong, 1978), or they may be unable objectively to identify students' strengths and weaknesses.

Burns (1982) links unsuccessful teaching to poor self-concept, stating that teachers who feel personally and professionally inadequate and who dislike teaching may be easily distracted and indifferent to pupil performance. Furthermore, they are predisposed to act in a hostile manner, tending to control the teaching situation.

As can be seen from Box 1.4, many of the features of successful teaching are linked to positive relationship skills; similarly, ineffective teacher behaviour is often linked to poor interpersonal skills and an inability to respect and value the student. Box 1.4 contrasts 14 features of the ineffective teacher with 14 identified features of the effective teacher.

BOX 1.4	*Fourteen traits of ineffective teachers contrasted with 14 traits of effective teachers*

Ineffective teacher traits	*Effective teacher traits*
Poor classroom management	Good role model
Poor relationship skills	Good interactive skills
Poor communicator	Good communicator
Lack of commitment	Enthusiastic
Plodding	Energetic
Self-conscious	Self-aware
Insensitive	Sensitive
Outspoken	Emotionally stable
Disruptive	Considerate
Disinterested	Curious
Distanced	Accessible
Threatening	Fair
Superior	Appropriate
Belittling	Encouraging

WHERE ARE YOU IN THE EFFECTIVE TEACHER – INEFFECTIVE TEACHER CONTINUUM?

Having read this brief review of the literature, you might be feeling that the good teacher has a wealth of characteristics that are beyond your grasp. Remember, however, that the good teacher is not perfect, and the good teacher has bad days. Nevertheless, teaching does benefit from analysis and reflection, and does improve with practice. There is plenty of room for all types of teacher, and, indeed, if you compare your ideas of good teaching with those of a colleague, you may both come up with very different types of ideal teacher – such variety is welcome. You may wish to consolidate this section by reading three articles from the recommended reading: Li (1997) and Benor and Leviyof (1997) offer two perspectives from other countries and make a good comparison with the UK system, whereas Davies et al (1996) discusses how nurse teachers can become more effective. All the studies are research based.

ACTIVITY 1.6	

At this point, take some time to reflect upon how many positive teaching characteristics you possess. Some things are difficult to change, such as intelligence and personality, but you should be able to develop and maximise your strengths when teaching, consciously practising the things you do well.

If you are concerned about your teaching skills, try to read the appropriate chapters in one of the books on communication style that are suggested in the further reading section at the end of the chapter. It may be helpful to focus on empathy, effective listening and questioning, exploring the use of such skills in your clinical work.

You may also find it helpful to develop a few ground rules to avoid falling into the ineffective teaching trap, for example:

- When giving a student feedback on her performance, always begin with the things that she has done well.
- Avoid pointing out errors or reprimanding in front of a patient, client or colleague.
- Call errors 'points to consider' rather than mistakes or weaknesses; try to focus on two or three major points, setting goals for improvement.
- Offer students your time: 'We could have 15 minutes this afternoon looking at this.'
- Always say when you do not know, and suggest ways of finding out.
- Observe the student sensitively and see if the response to 'How are you?' matches what you see. If not, explore further.

Finally, it is important that you develop a perceptive and objective self-concept. It is all too easy to evaluate a teaching session that you have just delivered in a negative way, focusing on the less good aspects, at the expense of celebrating the things you did well. If you genuinely value your own strengths, you will value what you see in others.

Although some people seem to be born teachers, the complexity of behaviours that constitute teaching can be learned and developed.

ACTIVITY 1.7

Write down one thing that you are good at as a teacher and that you would like to build upon.

You may be surprised at the strengths you possess. We will be referring to this later in the chapter, but meanwhile try to be aware of this aspect of your behaviour as you go about your work.

FACTORS AFFECTING LEARNING

Imagine the frustration of executing a perfect piece of cognitive teaching only to find that the learner is so anxious about getting her work done that she has been unable to attend to your session.

Child (1997) suggests that the teacher should consider cognitive entry characteristics in order to make an assessment of the student's or client's intellectual abilities. This is particularly important if someone is overwhelmed by the anxieties of a new ward or by the implications of a recently divulged diagnosis. It is also important to establish previous experience, determining whether or not the subject has been taught in the college or by a colleague, and exactly what the student knows about it. Similarly, it is important to find out just how much the patient/client knows so that you can build on this past experience to extend understanding and create new insights. Marson (1982) found that trainees often reported teaching experiences coming too soon to be assimilated as they lacked the necessary background knowledge and experience. Benner (1984) found that 'capturing' a patient's readiness to learn forms a key feature of effective teaching. Similarly, past experiences of teaching sessions may influence the students' perceptions of your role. Students may have had negative experiences that may interfere with your session until they realise that you have a different approach.

Communication skills (Child, 1997) are crucial in the teaching process. If your student has sensory impairment or limited vision or speech, you will have to be very sensitive with feedback to ensure that she is following and understanding.

Affective (i.e. emotional) characteristics will also impinge upon the teaching and learning process. The student's self-concept will influence the approach to learning. If she has recently been referred in an assessment or is repeatedly experiencing failure, she may believe herself to be incapable of the work and so block learning. Prompt feedback from you on successes, pinpointing areas on which she should concentrate in order to improve performance, will help the student to develop a more realistic self-concept.

Motivation influences learning, and this is strongly affected by the student's degree of interest. You can increase motivation in practice settings by helping the student to gain a sense of achievement as she integrates theory and practice. Motivation will be reduced, regardless of interest, if your teaching prevents the student from completing planned client care on time.

Anxiety may affect learning. Some of the best performances are undertaken in anxiety-provoking situations; however, if the degree of anxiety becomes intolerable, the student will be unable to learn. A student caring for an extremely sick patient may be able to improve care once you have provided a rationale for the various bits of equipment that she is expected to use, so she can see them in the context of the patient's care.

Personality may affect the process of learning. Marson (1982) found that personality clashes were a significant deterrent to learning. Moreover, someone who has an extroverted personality may enjoy sessions with distractions and digressions, whereas a more introverted person may be annoyed by these.

Embarrassment and discomfort may interfere with learning. The student who is taught or reprimanded in front of a client may fear that the client realises how little she knows; admitting you do not know can occasion discomfort and embarrassment. Similarly, a client may not wish to be taught in front of visitors.

Remember, too, that tiredness, pain, hunger or feeling unwell will all affect a person's ability to learn and develop. Atkinson et al (1996) provide an account of Piaget's stages of concept formation. The stages begin with sensorimotor at birth, move on next to iconic and then to concrete-symbolic at the age of 6 years, which is followed by formal and then finally post-formal at about 18 years of age. Biggs and Moore (1993) simplify the stages and explain them in a challenging way that can easily be applied to the education of adults. A person who is anxious, unwell or tired may move back (regress) to a stage of concept formation characteristic of a younger age group. To teach effectively, you may have to pitch your session in more concrete terms than you would have thought necessary, in order for clients or relatives to understand. If you discuss this with your colleagues, you may able to identify the factors that interfere with learning in your own students and take simple measures to minimise the effect of these. The key to doing this is to treat learners as adults (unless they patently are not), use negotiation, establish past cognitive and emotional experiences, and draw and build upon these, making clear links relevant to experience.

A FRAMEWORK FOR THE ANALYSIS OF TEACHING

Beattie's (1987) fourfold curriculum model (Fig. 1.1) provides a useful framework for the analysis of four different learning theories and four ways of structuring teaching. It is based on two axes. The vertical axis reflects definitions of knowledge, ranging from authoritative, consensual and closed (for example, facts that have been proved by research, such as the physiological events in the cardiac cycle), to knowledge that is conditional, reflexive and open (for example, the experience of conducting a first delivery, which has the potential to be different for every midwife). The horizontal axis places learning somewhere between intrinsic and extrinsic. The two axes form four boxes, which lend themselves to four different approaches to **curriculum** planning and, in our case, four ways of approaching learning and teaching, which we can now examine.

THE CURRICULUM AS A MAP OF KEY SUBJECTS

The curriculum as a map of key subjects would include a blend of biological, psychological, nursing, midwifery, medical and sociological sciences. In the practice setting, threads from these disciplines are drawn together to make the theory – practice link. These disciplines form the knowledge base that informs practice. For example, without an understanding of the physiology of the cardiovascular system, it would be difficult to give a patient who was being discharged on digitalis, effective and safe advice on taking the drug; similarly, a new mother

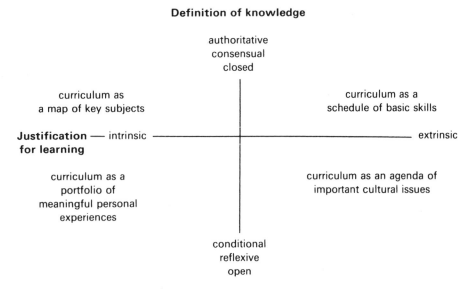

Figure 1.1 The fourfold curriculum (from Beattie 1987).

who wishes to breast-feed needs to be given information relating to her nutritional and fluid requirements.

In order to teach these subjects effectively, it is necessary to understand both the perceptual processes (see below) involved and **cognitive learning** theory. Cognitive learning theory emphasises active participation of the individual and the recognition of information in order to acquire complex information.

Perception

The **cognitive school of psychology** (practitioners of which believe that the mental processing of thoughts affects learning) suggest that learning can be stored in memory, retrieved and used in a new way when needed. Whatever the teacher intends the student to learn, the latter will make her own approximations according to the way in which she perceives stimuli and what she has already stored in memory from past experience and learning that is associated with what is being taught.

Followers of the **Gestalt school of psychology** talk about **perception** in relation to pattern perception. They describe four important features that make up the perceptual process. The principles of this process have great relevance to the way in which teachers structure their sessions.

The first principle is *similarity*. We need to form similar elements into a pattern of shape, size and colour. In teaching, we can use this principle by beginning with what the student knows. For example, a relative asks for an explanation of her brother's pleurisy and the symptoms he is experiencing. You ascertain that she has little knowledge of body function. You might begin by likening the pleura to a skirt with a petticoat underneath, the two layers gliding upon each other smoothly as the lungs move with breathing. The petticoat develops static electricity and the smooth movement of the layers is disturbed. You could move on to explain that the pleurae are sticking together, not because of static electricity but as a result of inflammation, that this prevents their free movement and that it is this fluid which is causing the pain. Analogies, then, have a useful place in enhancing perceptual processes.

Proximity, the second principle, refers to when similar objects appear close together and enhance accurate perception. In teaching, we could compare how alike one thing is to another, looking for similar and contrasting properties. Suppose you are teaching a student nurse or midwife the principles of wound management to enable her to care safely for patients/clients. You could begin by carrying out an aseptic technique on a patient or client with a small, sutured wound. Next, you could perform a dressing for a patient with a corrugated drain in situ, and then together you could check the vacuum on a closed drainage system. At the end of the morning, you would sit down together and look at the principles of care involved for the three patients/clients, comparing and contrasting the caring actions and emphasising the common principles of care.

Continuity occurs when similar parts of a figure, which appear in straight or curved lines, seem to stand out, so that the pattern is evident. Continuity can be achieved when teaching by following a theme with your student, by moving sequentially through a topic in a logical manner. As an example, a wife is getting ready for her husband's return home from hospital following a fractured spine, which has left him quadriplegic. Last week, a staff nurse taught her how to prevent constipation. Today, to achieve continuity, you are going to focus on ways of managing bowel evacuation, so your teaching is still linked to elimination needs, which you will ensure she understands, before moving on to discuss hygiene needs or their sexual relationship, for example.

The fourth principle is *closure*, which focuses on the fact that closed or partially closed figures are easier to perceive (the principle used in joining up the dots in children's comics). Thus, by closing a teaching session using a summary, or any other technique that allows integration of the material contained in the session, you will help the student to complete the perceptual pattern, tying all the threads together.

It is evident that by reflecting on how a learner organises information and by using these principles, we can make teaching more effective. If you wish to read more about perception, the chapter on this in Atkinson et al (1996) is enjoyable.

Learning by problem-solving

Myles (1993) describes how cognitive learning requires us to process the information received actively and transform it into new knowledge and categories. Its prerequisites are, therefore, the mental processes that perceive sensory inputs and the ability to encode it, store it in memory and retrieve it for later use.

Gestalt psychologists use the theory of insightful learning, which builds on the theory of perception. They describe insight as the sudden solution of a problem by perceiving the relationships essential to the solution. This may occasionally occur dramatically, and people often seek the experience of insight by completing crosswords, for example.

Kohler, a Gestalt psychologist, used chimpanzees to demonstrate the nature of problem-solving. Sultan, the chimp, is in a cage. Through the bars and out of reach is a piece of fruit; inside the cage is a short stick, and outside the cage, again out of reach, is a longer one. He tries to reach the fruit with the shorter of the two sticks and, frustrated, he tears at the netting. Next, there is a long pause while he gazes about him, scrutinising the area. Very purposefully now, the chimp uses the short stick to secure the larger stick, which he uses to reach the fruit. From the moment he begins the activity, his movements become one consecutive whole (Child, 1997). Sultan was also able to transfer this learning with the stick and was able to reach fruit hanging from the ceiling of his cage.

Trial and error learning may be evident at the beginning of problem-solving, but once the task is seen as a whole, it can be restructured in ways that affect solutions (Atkinson et al, 1996). The structure of the problem dictates the nature of problem-solving in Gestalt psychology. If a student is placed in a situation in which she has no knowledge, learning has to be by trial and error, and the patient on the receiving end of this may experience problems in his care of a more or less serious nature. Trial and error learning, then, may have its uses in a safe and controlled environment, but it is extremely unwise to risk this in the presence of a patient or client. Apart from basic safety, there are professional and legal issues if something goes wrong. If a student is presented with a problem for which it is possible to have a mental image, she may find a solution more easily.

Gestalt psychologists suggest that the efficiency of learning is dictated by the perceptual context in which learning takes place. They suggest that we learn by insight, using problem-solving.

Teaching by problem-solving

Myles (1993) refers to Fox (1975), who cites seven steps to problem-solving and links it to Kohler's experiment. Below, are the stages applied to helping a student to plan care.

1. *Problem*. A client who has been severely depressed following a stillbirth, but who is beginning to recover, asks to visit her baby's grave.
2. *Data collection*. Consider the situation and alternatives, her physical well-being, the motivation for the trip, her mood, the journey, etc.
3. *Hypothesis formulation*. A visit to her baby's grave would be therapeutic.
4. *Select plan for hypothesis testing*. What caring interventions may be necessary? Do you need medical consent? What if something goes wrong? Plan the journey (the what, where, when and hows).
5. *Test the hypothesis*. Implement the plan.
6. *Interpret the results*. It went well, the client returned looking tired yet relieved.
7. *Evaluate the hypothesis*. She has asked to go next time with a relative (so it is evident that the trip was therapeutic).

The student will have cared for a patient outside the security of the ward environment and will have developed insight into the detailed planning necessary for arranging such an activity.

The approach may look simplistic, and if it is, cognitive activity may have been minimal. Ornstein (1990) has some useful ideas for developing problem-solving skills, referring to Cybert's (1980) 10 steps (Box 1.5).

BOX 1.5	*Cybert's (1980) 10 steps to problem-solving*

1. Keep the basic problem in mind and avoid distractions. In the example given, you may need to forget problems of staffing, pressures of ward routine, etc.
2. Avoid early commitment to a hypothesis
3. Simplify the problem by using phrases, symbols or formulae
4. Change an approach as soon as you can see that it is not working
5. Ask questions and attempt to answer them
6. Be willing to question assumptions
7. Work backwards, if necessary, to work out solutions
8. Keep in mind practical solutions that may later be combined
9. Use analogies (when you draw similarities between two things, for example, referring to the similarities between a skirt and its petticoat, and the layers of the pleura)
10. Talk about the problem

This approach moves problem-solving away from the realm of a superficial guessing game and provides a structured framework within which it can take place.

Before you can begin problem-solving, the learner needs relevant information in order to assess the situation. In the example described, this may be a knowledge of the effects of depression and grieving, an awareness of drug interactions, the client's history, etc., which will form the prerequisite information. The more able you are to help the learner set the problem in context, using concrete examples, the better able she will be to solve the problem. Having solved the problem, you may then help the learner to apply concepts ('This worked for Mrs Green, what about Mr Brown?') so that she is able to generalise and adapt her professional practice.

ACTIVITY 1.8

Now try out this approach for yourself. In the group of clients for whom you and a learner are caring, identify a client problem that is fairly common, albeit for a variety of reasons, for example, difficulties with breathing, slow wound healing or poor self-image. Select one patient/client for whom this problem is a priority.

State the problem.

1. What information does the student need in order to work out solutions? Are there any exceptional or irregular circumstances to be taken into account?

2. Use questions to draw on the student's knowledge base, and be ready to develop insight by offering explanations (**exposition**). Note below the key questions you might use.

3. Help the student to collect all the relevant information that she needs in order to state the problem (care plans, drug charts, text books, etc.).

4. **Brainstorm** (without evaluating) with the student, as many possible solutions that you can think of, writing them down as they come to mind.

5. In the light of the student's knowledge base:
   - evaluate each idea
   - challenge
   - question and seek a rationale
   - ask for limits and constraints for the range of alternatives
   - select the most feasible solution.

6. Plan jointly how to implement this.

7. Implement the plan. If it has not materialised as envisaged, return to stage 3 of this activity.

8. Evaluate the process together.

9. Ask the student to examine the appropriateness of the chosen intervention with other clients who have the same problem in order to establish whether the solution is open to generalisation.

Undertaking an exercise of this kind clearly requires that you are able to work with the student for a span of duty in order to complete the suggested process.

Problem-solving is an easy exercise if it takes place at a superficial level; to achieve depth poses a greater challenge. You may need to use the technique yourself several times in order to get it right and become familiar and comfortable with it.

Teaching by using an advanced organiser

Ausubel, an educational psychologist, developed the notion of an advanced organiser to complement his theory that learning occurs through the interaction of new material with information already stored in memory (Myles, 1993).

The advanced organiser is an introductory statement of a high degree of depth that is broad enough to encompass all the information that will follow in the session (Myles, 1987). Its purpose is to give students the information they need to understand the session, that is, it will help to 'create set'. The organiser will also bring to mind information that the student already has that she may have thought irrelevant to the session. In this way, the bridge is built between existing information and new material.

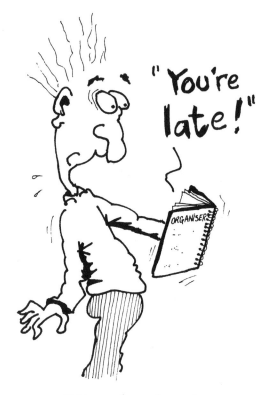

Using an advanced organiser

In order for learning to occur in a meaningful way, three factors have to be considered. First, the student must have an appropriate learning set, that is, a readiness to learn in a certain way. Second, the new material must have logical meaning, so that it can be related to the student's own cognitive structures in order to provide the foundations on which to build new material. Finally, the student's own cognitive structures (memory) must contain specifically relevant ideas so that new information can be integrated with it. Consideration of these three factors will mean that the teacher begins at the right level (Quinn, 1995).

In this way, new ideas are not just added to the pile of old learning but instead become integrated with existing knowledge, skills or attitudes to form a new cognitive structure with greater meaning (Quinn, 1995).

Ausubel's model is appropriate for teaching in the practice setting since it builds upon the involvement between student and teacher, makes use of examples and uses deductive reasoning (knowledge gained by working things out). Finally, the model is sequential, beginning with an advanced organiser that links existing knowledge to new by forming conceptual bridges (Myles, 1993). Ausubel believes there is a parallel between the organisation of subject matter by the teacher and the way in which people organise knowledge in their minds, that is, their information-processing system.

The model has three phases of activity: first, the presentation of an advanced organiser; second, the presentation of the learning task; and finally, the strengthening of the cognitive organisation (Joyce and Weil, 1986).

The advanced organiser can be presented in several forms: expository, comparative (Joyce and Weil, 1986) and diagrammatic (Myles, 1987).

Take the example of a practice nurse setting up a slimming group for clients. The aim of her first meeting is to generate motivation to lose weight by explaining the effects that obesity has upon an individual. The advanced organiser could be as shown in Figure 1.2. The subject matter may be organised with the use of a film, leaflets and group work.

The organiser is at a higher level of abstraction and inclusiveness than the learning itself, in that it explains, integrates and interrelates the material in the learning task with previously learned material (Joyce and Weil, 1986, p.76), so it provides pegs on which to hang the material that follows. The teacher, then, must help to explore the organiser as well as the subsequent learning. For example, in the slimming group, the teacher will have to explain why different diseases result from being overweight. She may ask members what happens to their breathing if they run or climb stairs, and clients may disclose the medical problems they experience.

The learning task may involve explanations of energy intake and output, and the introduction of a healthy eating plan that is restricted in saturated fats, together with encouraging graded exercises.

To end the session and strengthen the cognitive organisation, the nurse may emphasise the importance of weight loss by revising the hazards of obesity, stressing that it is not too late to prevent further damage. She would ask students to summarise the key principles of the diet and exercise plan, repeating definitions and asking for differences between aspects of the regime.

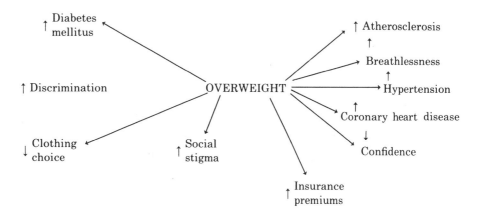

Figure 1.2 Example of an advanced organiser.

ACTIVITY 1.9

Think of one topic or theme that is frequently taught in your clinical area. Make an advanced organiser for this and outline how the session would evolve. You may find this quite hard to do. Practice will help you to develop this method, but you need also to check that your lesson plan matches the organiser and that unintroduced material does not appear.

This section has looked at the curriculum as a map of key subjects, examining how students learn and suggesting teaching approaches that will enable such learning to take place. It is crucial in this type of learning and teaching to build on the student's existing knowledge base.

Teaching strategies that are appropriate for use within the four models include exposition (providing chunks of explanation), the use of questions and answers, guided study with feedback, crosswords and quizzes, handouts (both written and diagrammatic), the use of case studies, buzz groups, **brainstorming** and problem-solving.

Regardless of your practice setting, you should be able to build up a resource bank of visual aids to support your teaching, including textbooks, research papers and journal articles, diagrams, models and items of disposable equipment, in addition to mental models such as analogies. Finally, the value of the patient/client and of your own experience, in teaching, cannot be underestimated.

THE CURRICULUM AS A SCHEDULE OF BASIC SKILLS

This aspect of the curriculum is described by Beattie (1987, p. 20) as those areas of practical competence which are 'deemed to be essential for responsible and effective performance of professional tasks'.

In every clinical area there are skills that are either specific to that area or general to many placements. A complex matrix can be devised illustrating the skills a student needs to achieve the competencies, against the **psychomotor skills** that are specific to the clinical context.

In terms of patient/client teaching, there may be skills that either a carer or the client has to be able to carry out in order to be discharged into the community. For example, a person with diabetes needs to be able to measure the glucose concentration of his blood, give insulin injections correctly, etc. A client with learning difficulties will have to master daily living activities such as dressing and making drinks, while a carer may need to manage emotional outbursts and unpredictable behaviour patterns. A new mother needs to feel confident in caring for her baby on a day-to-day level, managing baths and feeds. A client who is confused needs to be able to administer his own medication safely.

Learning from behavioural theories

These theories focus on the deliberate shaping of behaviour towards a desired goal. The **behavioural** school of psychology argues that the role played by the environment is crucial to learning. If the environment is structured correctly, learning will occur regardless of the volition of the teacher, as connections are made between **stimulus** and **response**, and response and **reinforcement**.

Myles (1993) identifies three 'key tenets' that form the basis of behavioural psychology:

1. contiguity
2. classical conditioning
3. operant conditioning.

Contiguity refers to the situation in which, if two events repeatedly occur together, they will later become associated, so that when only one event is present, the other will be remembered (that is, the stimulus evokes a response). Myles stresses the significance of this in nursing when teaching and practising psychomotor skills: in order that the correct sequence is always followed, the teacher should not encourage the repetition of inappropriate responses when someone is demonstrating a skill, as this destroys contiguity. Contiguity can be achieved by teaching skills in a systematic way.

Classical conditioning, made famous by Pavlov in the 1920s, focuses upon achieving certain reflexive responses by using stimuli. His famous experiment in which dogs were conditioned to salivate at the sound of a bell is an example of this. Myles (1993) suggests that this theory has little place in teaching, although original accounts of this work make interesting reading.

Operant conditioning, however, is a behavioural process that brings about purposeful actions. In this process, the animal (learner) is active and behaviour brings about important consequences. Skinner is famous for his work in this field. In his experiments, a hungry rat is placed in a 'Skinner' box, which contains a bar with a food box beneath it. As the rat explores his new environment, he occasionally presses the bar; every time he does this, to his pleasure, a food pellet is delivered. This reward dramatically increases the incidence of bar pressing. If the food reward is not given, the operant response (bar-pressing) undergoes extinction. However, if a pattern of partial reinforcement is used, the extinction of operant behaviour is usually much slower. There are important principles here for teaching: first, if random behaviour is rewarded consistently, the incidence of that behaviour will increase; second, partial reinforcement delays extinction; and third, if behaviour is not rewarded (ignored), it is extinguished, a useful guideline for managing unwanted behaviour.

These principles can be applied to the child who has tantrums. If the parents occasionally reinforce this by giving in to whatever the child demands, they will receive more persistent outbursts than the parent who invariably gives way; while those who consistently hold out and refuse the demands enjoy the absence of such behaviour.

Operant conditioning plays an important part in the learning of new processes. Many driving instructors are expert in this approach. Behaviour is often shaped by positively reinforcing the subject as the behaviour gets nearer and nearer the desired response, for example, reversing efficiently or changing gear smoothly, by using phrases such as 'much better' or 'nearly there'.

It is important to consider the set of rewards that you would wish to give. Some of you may have experience of caring for clients using behavioural regimes, which reward positive or newly taught behaviour. In teaching, social reinforcers are usually used; these include nods, smiles, praise, eye contact, writing students' responses down and the verbal reinforcers of 'well done', etc.

The concept of punishment (although of little value in clinical teaching practice) is an interesting issue; teachers punish using put-downs and sarcasm and by keeping students at a distance. Punishment decreases the probability of a response, but it fails to give the learner an alternative choice of behaviour. The effects on the learner of the use of punishment can be worry, dislike of the punisher and deviant behaviour.

Teaching using behavioural theories

Many of you who work with clients who require a high degree of skilled teaching (such as children or those with learning difficulties) will be expert in this field. Behavioural principles were used 20 or more years ago to underpin the trend for programmed learning, which has now gone out of fashion, to be replaced by computer-assisted learning (CAL). There are several teaching principles that emerge from this theory:

- Each step in the learning process should be short and grow out of previously learned behaviours so that the stages of a skill are broken down and linked.
- Learning should be regularly rewarded and carefully controlled by continuous or intermittent reinforcement (Child, 1997). When teaching, you may move through a continuum from continuous to intermittent reinforcement. Social reinforcers, used in a variable ratio, are very positively received, and rapid feedback on a student's work will promote learning. Something as simple as 'You cared well for Mrs Jones this morning; she looks comfortable' has enormous potential as a reinforcer. Reinforcement can be used in this way to 'shape' behaviour. Shaping is an important concept. A shy student who has been allocated to your unit and receives positive reinforcement as she adopts the **group norms** is likely to settle quickly into her role. The principle of extinction may be useful if a student or client is displaying undesirable behaviour; ignoring the event serves to make it non-profitable, especially if acceptable behaviour is rewarded.
- The reward should follow immediately after the desired response appears (Child, 1997). Although this has been briefly mentioned above, in true behaviourism, a delayed reward is meaningless as the reinforcement will not be linked to the operant behaviour.

Teaching using simulations

Some 30 years ago, simulation had a high profile in professional education, with a large practical classroom in every school of nursing or midwifery that could be turned into an operating theatre or delivery room in minutes. Some of the more mature readers of this chapter may have been deemed fit to practice as the result of an examination conducted as a simulation.

Nowadays, simulations can be very sophisticated, often taking place in a skills laboratory, relying on computer technology, which can represent anything from the flight deck of an aircraft to wind-surfing. Similarly, situations may be enacted using board games, for example, Monopoly simulating 'real-estate speculation'; Joyce and Weil, 1986). Conducting a simulation requires forethought so that you have time to devise a game, or collect together the equipment, including any software that you might need. Skills laboratories allow for the simulation of practice in a safe environment and may provide an arena for trial and error learning with feedback.

The simulation model rests upon the principles of cybernetics, essentially a feedback system, which generates movement towards a desired goal, monitors errors and redirects behaviour. The recent craze for virtual pets is an excellent example of this.

A simulation has the advantage of making the learning task less complex than when it occurs in the real world. For example, once the position of a proposed stoma has been decided, nurses can begin preoperatively to teach a patient how to use appliances and manipulate equipment, establishing the best positions and practising without the hazards of a wound, drain site or intravenous infusion and all the postoperative discomforts. Similarly, students may 'fumble' with equipment on a resuscitation trolley before they have to use it for real.

In a simulation, the student learns from direct self-generated feedback on crashing the plane or stalling the engine. In the simulations described in this chapter, the student may need teaching help with feedback as awareness and perception are not enhanced in a simulation (Joyce and Weil, 1986). It is the principles of behaviourism, rather than cognitive learning, that direct the student.

Within a simulation exercise, the role of the teacher is very important; because the student is so involved in practising the skill of the simulation, she may not be aware of what she is learning and experiencing. The teacher needs to bring the concepts and principles underpinning the simulation to the forefront of the student's mind and to elicit her reactions. Thus, when teaching the patient stoma management, you may wish the patient to experience running around, lying or sitting with a full bag, with it pulling away from the skin. You will stress that, in the real world, the consistency of the stool will be different but the weight will be the same. You may then explore feelings, anxieties, the cosmetic effect on appearance, etc. In midwifery, you may demonstrate a bath using a doll so that the procedure is learned in the absence of a wet, wriggling baby.

In psychiatry, a carer may wish to **role play** a strategy that she intends to use with a client. For example, she may wish to confront a woman whom she believes has alcohol hidden on the ward. The simulation will allow her to check out and modify her tactics. Similarly, if the simulation revolves around a game, the rules of the game need to be spelled out and be on hand for checking.

If a team approach is used in a simulation, the teacher may need to act as a referee. Additionally, activities such as coaching, offering advice, supporting or suggesting the way forward are all appropriate within this model.

Finally, once the simulation is completed, the teacher needs to create an awareness of the difficulties that may arise when using this exercise in a real situation (Joyce and Weil, 1986). The student will learn from the direct result of the simulation and, additionally and importantly, as a result of teaching interventions.

A simulation has four phases that guide lesson planning (Joyce and Weil, 1986):

1. *Orientation*. Outline the topic and concepts to be incorporated into the activity and present an overview of the simulation.
2. *Participant training*. Practise the skill.
3. *Simulation*. Then give feedback, evaluate and clarify any misconceptions.
4. *Debriefing*. Summarise events and perceptions, examine difficulties and insights, analyse the processes involved, compare the simulation with real life and relate it to clinical experiences or to the clients' expected progress.

Joyce and Weil (1986) suggest that the use of a simulation has the potential to create a sense of effectiveness, enabling people to face consequences, and encourage an increase in knowledge, empathy, critical thinking, decision-making and, finally, concepts and skills.

ACTIVITY 1.10

Below, we have given you space to plan a simulation to use in your own work environment, for example baby-bathing, helping a client to cook a meal, scrubbing up and assisting a surgeon, assembling and using resuscitation equipment, rehearsing reminiscence therapy or helping a client to express breast milk.

1. What activity do you intend to simulate? Note your intention in doing this and any equipment, visual aids and resources that you will need. Remember that you need to cite here details of the environment that will be suitable for conducting the simulation.

2. Note key points for the orientation phase.

3. Outline the details of the participant training (a **skills analysis**) by breaking down the procedure into small steps.

4. Conduct the simulation, noting the key points for the next stage.

5. Debrief: What did you learn from the exercise?

6. Evaluate: Does the session need modifying?

Once you have completed the six stages, you have a workable plan that can be used over and over again, perhaps with some minor modifications as the situation differs.

Teaching using social learning theory

Social learning theory can be considered as a behavioural approach, although it overlaps to a certain extent with the domain of cognitive psychology.

Vicarious learning (when you do not realise you have learned until you need to demonstrate the behaviour) is also a feature of social learning theory and is defined as 'learning by watching the behaviour of others and observing what consequences it produces for them' (Atkinson et al, 1996). Learning by modelling (this being planned and conscious) views behaviour as a two-way interaction between an individual and his environment. Complex patterns of behaviour can be acquired in this way (Quinn, 1995). Myles (1993) believes that emotional responses can also be learned by modelling. At the beginning of the chapter, we asked you to identify the characteristics of an effective teacher. If you described a positive role model, she may be responsible for an enormous amount of vicarious learning on your part.

Bandura (1977) describes four features of the model and observer (Box 1.6).

Research indicates that the most influential models are seen by the learner as having status, power and prestige (Myles, 1993). Myles also reminds us of nursing research that indicates how strongly nurses are influenced by colleagues, especially the ward sister (Fretwell, 1982; Melia, 1983). He makes two important recommendations that incorporate the principles of social learning. The first is the maintenance of high professional standards; the second is that teachers should only model behaviour that they would wish others to

| BOX 1.6 | *Bandura's (1977) features of the model and observer* |

- *Attentional processes,* that is, the degree of interpersonal attraction (liking) between the model and observer, and how useful and distinctive the observed behaviour is. The frequency of contact with the model affects the adoption of the behaviour; similarly, the observer's level of arousal and ability to process information will determine what is learned. Finally, learning will also be influenced by perceptual set (what the observer expects to see) and the amount of previous reinforcement.
- *The retention process* is the second characteristic of this model. Remembering the modelled behaviour is a crucial aspect of learning; **rehearsal** and repetition are therefore important elements.
- *The model has a motor reproduction phase,* that is, the student enacts the observed behaviour and evaluates it in terms of accuracy.
- *Motivation affects learning:* the behaviour is likely to be learned if there is value in it and it has meaning for the learner.

adopt. Much of the teaching that you do in this category may occur without your awareness. However, there are ways in which you can build up Bandura's principles, which the following example will demonstrate.

A student comes to you to report that, during the morning, a patient, on a unit caring for older people, has been weeping. This is quite unusual as the gentleman is making a good recovery and is almost ready to go home. The student feels that she is unable to meet his needs and asks for your help.

In terms of attentional processes, together you evaluate the situation and agree that the patient needs time to talk and express his distress. With the student, you plan how this can be facilitated. Using the question and answer technique (described in Chapter 6), you help the student to revise the verbal and non-verbal strategies that indicate listening and which will help the patient to talk.

As you run through each strategy, you note a key word on a sheet of paper so that the student has access to it during the interaction. Then encourage the student to observe you closely, noting how you use the strategies you have written down, and ask her to note those behaviours you use which enhance the interaction and those which might inhibit it. Encourage her to write these down, as well as any questions she may think of when at the bedside. The student is then cued, that is, she is given a series of prompts. As far as possible, you may rehearse by running through again the strategies you intend to use and then carry out the planned care.

To activate retentional processes, you establish whether or not you found the cause of this gentleman's distress. You then ask the student to identify the strategies you used and evaluate their effectiveness, underlining each tactic on her handout as she mentions it and writing an example of each under the heading. You may also look for behaviours that inhibited the interaction and discuss ways of minimising the effect of these.

To achieve motor reproduction, you ask the student to select two strategies from the list that she would like to develop. You then plan an interaction with a different client, with the student initiating listening behaviours and you acting as observer or resource if needed. Together, you then evaluate her performance, away from the client.

Motivational processes can be activated by reinforcing the success of her interaction, explaining the difference that the interaction has made to the perception of the patient and consequently his care. You may help the student to identify a skill in listening that she has the potential to develop further.

The teaching and learning behaviours that exist within the model of the curriculum as 'a schedule of basic skills' are not the narrow field of activities that one might initially expect. Principles from this area lend themselves to teaching how to tie a shoelace, at one end of the spectrum, to assertion at the other. The strategies you might adopt include demonstration, supervised practice, simulation and role modelling.

THE CURRICULUM AS AN AGENDA OF IMPORTANT CULTURAL ISSUES

Viewing the curriculum as an agenda of important cultural issues helps us to focus on teaching about both long-and short-term dilemmas and controversies in practice, and may include both practical and ethical debates. I am sure that, in your working environment, you can identify many issues that fit into this category. Similarly, clients or patients may need to be aware of issues surrounding choices they may make, for example, with respect to treatment, such as consent to drug therapy or induction of labour, organ donation or HIV testing.

The teaching emphasis in this category is both social and democratic in that students may work in groups to raise awareness of issues that may have no easy solution. The teacher needs a high level of interpersonal skills to facilitate such sessions.

Teaching using a group investigation model

The model is based on democratic processes and group decisions (Joyce and Weil, 1986). It stimulates enquiry in an atmosphere of reason and negotiation as the students together try to work through problems and seek answers.

The teacher plays a facilitative role, focusing primarily on the group process, perhaps helping the students to formulate a plan, while acting as a source of knowledge and resources, and keeping the project within manageable boundaries.

If you are studying this chapter as one of a peer group, you will be able to engage in the next activity. If you are studying alone, the next exercise will not be possible but may be something that you are able to refer back to. The structure of the model is applied in the following activity.

ACTIVITY 1.11

With your student group, select an issue that is pertinent to practice, such as the problem of gaining informed consent in emergency situations. Think of an example from your own practice area since it is important that this activity be carried out with real benefit to your area and the staff involved.

1. Plan a short teaching session to explain the complexities of the situation so that all aspects of the situation are outlined.

2. Explore the reactions to the situation and note these on a flip chart. (Keep a separate record of these.)

3. With the group, decide on ways in which the issue can be explored and organise how information will be collected. For example, one student may go to the library to look for definitions, two students may design and issue short questionnaires to patients, and one student may interview medical staff.

4. Allocate deadlines for this material to be collected.

5. At the next session, as the group members present material and ask questions, challenge the students to find their own answers.

6. Recycle the activity. Does a new problem or activity emerge (Joyce and Weil, 1986)? If, for example, informed consent has to be pursued, it may be that you now need to consider the significance of how this is documented in your records.

You may have found the six steps demanding in allowing students freedom to explore and debate. Note here the behaviours that you were aware you used that enabled the process to take place.

The model may be one that is difficult to plan ahead for, since relevant situations tend to emerge without warning. However, this is not always the case.

Joyce and Weil (1986) suggest the model can teach cognitive knowledge as well as social processes. Additionally, such sessions provide a medium for fostering interpersonal relationships in the team as well as independence in learning and respect for the views of others.

The facilitator in such a model needs to have a knowledge of and access to varied resources. For example, you may know of key research reports or journal articles, or be able to introduce the group to appropriate personnel who have access to information. Your negotiated role may be to invite an expert speaker who can offer a perspective on an issue the group is exploring; for example, the chaplain may have relevant resources, or you may have a colleague with a philosophy degree who could help with an ethical dilemma.

The curriculum, as an agenda of important cultural issues, relies on the teacher facilitating the exploration of uncertainties. The learning group may be students, clients in a support group, the multidisciplinary team, relatives or carers. Teaching methods may include projects, **syndicates**, case discussion or the use of **critical incident analysis**.

THE CURRICULUM AS A PORTFOLIO OF MEANINGFUL PERSONAL EXPERIENCES

The distinction between personal and social learning is blurred, and you may well come to the conclusion that the concepts and principles embedded within each category influence and affect each other. Beattie (1987) describes a 'portfolio of meaningful personal experiences' as being organised around the individual student's interests and needs. The intention is that the student will reflect upon practice and share the experience with others. Beattie goes on to describe how it can be used for professional, moral and personal encounters. Similarly, for the patient or client, it may be an opportunity to explore the context of illness. The wife of a client diagnosed as schizophrenic, for example, may wish to explore the role of the charity MIND and take an active part in its work so that she, too, is doing something that may promote awareness. She may need your skills to help her reflect on this role in a purposeful way. You might imagine a similar situation with the new parents of a baby with Down's syndrome.

Benner (1984) highlights the importance of reflection in her research, which uses the Dreyfus model of skill acquisition to demonstrate how students pass through five levels of 'proficiency' ranging from novice to expert. Benner's work clearly indicates the problem of the theory – practice gap and is essential reading for anyone wishing to develop a teaching role in the practice setting.

The *novice* moves to a ward after a period in college, learning 'the rules' and principles of basic skills. These rules are inflexible, and novice students are unable to contextualise them, that is, they are unable to make small adjustments to skills in order to apply them in practice.

The '*advanced beginner*' demonstrates a 'marginally acceptable performance'. Benner states that a mentor may have helped her to cope with sufficient situations, issuing guidelines, to enable the student to apply the rules.

The *competent practitioner* will have been in her role for 2 years or more; she is consciously aware of her actions and has a feeling of mastery but lacks the speed and flexibility of the proficient nurse. Benner suggests that a mentor can enhance practice by using decision-making games and simulations that help the student to plan and coordinate complex care situations.

The *proficient nurse* has a deep understanding of the situation, in that she experiences it as similar to a past experience stored in memory, and in this way, a plan develops unconsciously.

The *expert* has an intuitive grasp of each situation and is able to select and analyse a problem without consideration of the alternative aspects. An example is a ward manager who, seemingly intuitively, advises the night staff to watch a patient closely and predicts a sudden change in condition, which materialises.

Schön (1987) would contend that personalising and reflecting upon experiences enables the student to transfer professional knowledge to 'real world practices', enabling the student to progress through Benner's five stages. Schön discusses at length the notion of professional artistry, calling it a form of intelligence, a kind of knowing, although different from professional knowledge. Artistry is demonstrated when competent practice is displayed in conflicting situations.

Schön (1987) calls this 'knowing-in-action'. He contends that 'reflection-in-action' will develop this professional artistry so that a bridge is built between theory and practice. You may remember, at the beginning of this chapter, that teaching was defined as an art, purposefully within this context. Reflection, then, is something that you can facilitate in others and develop in yourself. Do read Bolt's (1991) work on *Becoming Reflective*.

Learning through personal growth

This approach to learning is largely based on the influential and classic work of Rogers (1983), who holds that education should 'facilitate the process of change in an individual so that she or he may function fully'. This is called a **humanistic** approach, in which the belief is that individuals are free to choose their own direction.

Rogers developed his ideas from his work in non-directive counselling; the approach is based on the assumption that learning is a development of self. Assuming that every individual has the potential for self-development, the facilitator attempts to reduce the differences in level of knowledge from what is known towards the aspired level, which will help the client to sort out his problems.

Rogers stresses the importance of the tutor–student relationship in which the student explores ideas about work and relationships with others and achieves personal integration, effectiveness and realistic self-appraisal (Joyce and Weil, 1986). The approach depends upon students taking responsibility for their own learning.

Joyce and Weil summarise the key features of the humanistic approach:

1. Individuals have a natural drive to learn.
2. Learning can be maximised by using experience.
3. Self-evaluation encourages independence and creativity.

In order to bring about this type of teaching, Joyce and Weil suggest that the facilitator needs skills in building a lasting, non-threatening relationship, for example, in:

■ listening and responding consistently
■ helping the student to identify feelings and personal knowledge
■ sharing of herself
■ being sensitive to the student's needs
■ being aware of personal strengths and weaknesses and the effect upon others. This has links with Burns' concept of the effective teacher discussed earlier in the chapter.

Rogers tends to make the practice of such a style sound easy. As with other models, the development of this approach takes time and practice, and the adoption of such a stand requires considerable reflection and personal development on the part of the teacher.

Teaching from a student's experience

Miles (1987) describes how the teacher can build upon the experiences of the student, using an experiential learning cycle. This can form a useful framework for maximising teaching in practice settings (Fig. 1.3).

An example of how the model might be used is when a 'novice' (Benner, 1984) is caring for patients before and after gynaecological surgery. As a teacher, you are trying to help her apply the rules of pre- and postoperative care to a particular patient, planning care for a patient who is to have an abdominal hysterectomy. The patient is resting after premedication, and you sit down with the student to explain the nature of the operation, using a labelled diagram. Together, you escort the patient to theatre and remain with her during anaesthetic induction. The student remains in theatre, shadowing the charge nurse to observe the operation and to monitor the care given in the initial stages of recovery.

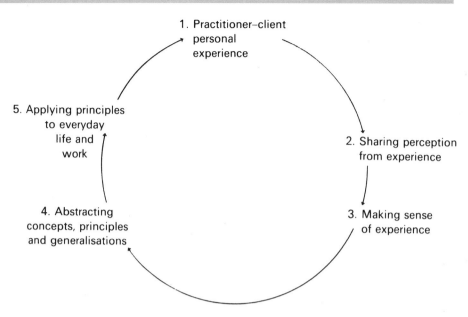

Figure 1.3 An experiential learning cycle (Adapted from Miles 1987).

Once the patient is back in bed and her immediate needs have been met, you encourage the student to share her perceptions of her experience, perhaps with the other students on the ward. You may ask what she saw and felt. Initially, the student may be overwhelmed by her initiation into the theatre environment: incisions, blood, smells, the beauty of the pelvic organs. She may, however, go on to describe how brutal retractors are. She may, with your prompting, recall the surgical procedure. As she talks, you write her perceptions down on a large sheet of paper using key words.

In order to make sense of the experience, the student needs to understand what it all means so that she can transfer all this to inform (that is, to illuminate) future postoperative nursing care. You revisit the key words on the flip chart, for example 'retractors', encouraging the student to work out the effect that this has on the patient. She may identify bruising or stretching, and you may then be able to demonstrate how this contributes to pain, discussing how the potential problems could be managed. Abstracting concepts, generalisations and principles may be achieved by exploring the extent to which the other patients in your client group who have had a hysterectomy have experienced similarities and differences in their needs and planned nursing care.

The example given is concrete. The experience could, with equal validity, be the administration of the student's first injection, the first experience of induced labour, breaking bad news or handling an emotional outburst. What is important is that the student agrees to the use of her experience for teaching purposes.

The potential of the model for client teaching is varied. Consider the person with newly diagnosed diabetes who is to have a hypoglycaemic attack induced so that the person and his family can recognise and manage the situation when it occurs. First, the patient and relatives should be prepared by explaining what to expect. The hypoglycaemic attack is induced, and the patient is stabilised.

You explore with both parties what was observed and what was felt. You are then in a position to make sense of the experience by linking what happened to altered physiology. From this, you can deduce the features of a hypoglycaemic attack and how to manage it, deriving concepts and principles. Finally, you apply the principles to everyday life – coping with exercise, etc.

Teaching through a reflective process

Boud et al (1985) describe a process that develops the learning experience using a reflective cycle (Fig. 1.4). The model has three phases: the experience, the reflective process and the outcomes.

The student, client or colleague identifies an experience that she wishes to explore with you. She should be asked to reflect on the experience and to record the salient points, that is, to replay the events. This account could be a verbal, written or visual exploration. The next step is to ask the student to focus on the feelings associated with the experience in order to use positive emotions and to examine, remove or balance the effects of negative feelings. In re-evaluating the experience, a re-examination of events in the light of reflection takes place to cement the learning that has occurred.

Let us take the following example to demonstrate the technique. A client, adapting to life in a self-propelled wheelchair, takes himself off to 'have a go' in the streets surrounding the hospital. On his return to the ward, over a much-needed coffee, the two of you reflect on the process.

You begin by asking what happened. The client describes the positive side of his outing but states that he will only use the chair in his garden. It transpires that a well-meaning pedestrian, without invitation, propelled the patient across a pedestrian crossing, thus disempowering him. Feelings such as anger, helplessness and embarrassment emerge. The client may be laughing or crying as his emotions are released. You may help him to put his emotions in perspective by exploring how real they are. Who was staring? Was the pusher patronising or concerned? The client should be helped to see that he did achieve his objective and, if it is appropriate, be helped to alter his perception. Importantly, you could help the client to identify strategies that would deter offers of unwanted

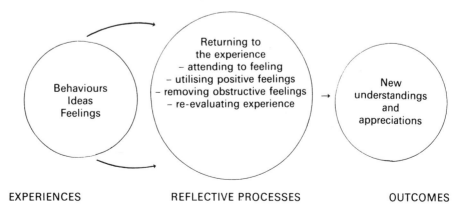

Figure 1.4 The reflective cycle (After Boud et al 1985).

help. In rehearsing some of these, he could judge their effects upon the would-be helper, and in this way new outcomes to the situation might emerge. If the client does not work through his negative emotions, he will not adapt to the full extent of his potential.

Schön (1987) states that reflection helps others to make decisions in conditions of uncertainty. He suggests two ways of reflecting: first, by thinking back on an action, as described; and second, by stopping before or mid-action to think and generate a different outcome. In this way, professional and personal behaviour will become shaped and reshaped. If you think it necessary to stop a student in mid-action, do so, but execute this away from the patient so that the student maintains her poise and the patient is unaware of any potential problem.

ACTIVITY 1.12

1. At the beginning of this chapter, you identified some of your strengths as teacher. Select a teaching session that you have undertaken in the past week. Write an account of the session. Pay close attention to detail, noting events that occurred and your reactions. Include recollections of judgements you made at the time, but try not to interpret your story just yet.

2. List the emotions and thoughts that you have about the session. Select the positive ideas and consider ways of maximising them in other teaching sessions. Now examine the negative feelings you may have. To change your perspective, imagine that, in your place, someone whom you think of as a good role model carries out your session in exactly the same way. She invites you to discuss her negative emotions. What interpretations would you put on them?

3. Consider ways of incorporating strategies into your lesson plan that will minimise these negative aspects in your next session.

You will undoubtedly have found this exercise difficult to do at anything other than a superficial level unless you are comfortable with self-reflection. Practice reflection and it will become a habit. Reflection may be developed by writing a reflective journal, as described in Chapter 6, perhaps by focusing upon aspects of your role, such as assertion or counselling skills, that you wish to develop.

Valuable personal experiences can be created in groups or in one-to-one settings. You may discover a large overlap in this area with teaching that occurs socially, that is, using the group investigation model.

While learning through reflection is a powerful medium, like all methods, it has its pitfalls. Within this type of work, Rich and Parker (1995) point out the ethical and moral dilemmas that may arise from such work; this article is listed in the further reading section and will help you to balance the advantages with the pitfalls before you jump on the bandwagon.

Methods that help the student to learn and develop from reflective practice include reflection itself, the numerous activities that make up experiential learning, critical incident analysis, problem-solving, journal writing, video feedback, **process recordings** and discussion.

TEACHING AND LEARNING USING THE FOURFOLD CURRICULUM

Figure 1.5 plots the four ways of approaching teaching that complement Beattie's (1986) four ways of viewing learning opportunities for any learner in your working environment. If you have completed the activities, you will now have lesson plans for each of the four approaches, which you can use as a model for other sessions.

ACTIVITY 1.13

Compare and contrast the four styles of lesson plan. What are the difficulties and strengths of each approach? How do the role of teacher and learner change with each type? How comfortable are you with these roles? You may discover that you are able to switch categories or that your work and style suit just one or two.

By now, you will have realised that principles of behaviourism enter into your cognitive learning session as you smile, nod and value student contributions; cognitive strategies have crept into your skills teaching; personal and social learning strategies have fused together, personal learning enhancing cognitive teaching, so that the knowledge gained from each session interacts with, relates to and complements learning in the other three areas.

You may wish to reflect upon the methods you use most frequently, investing some time in studying the uses and abuses of all the different methods you could employ, ranging from teacher led to student centred (Sheahan, 1980).

How can you devise a teaching and learning programme in your area that meets the four requirements of the map of key subjects: a schedule of basic skills, a portfolio of meaningful personal experiences and an agenda of important cultural issues? You may already have identified learning objectives for students that work in your area. Many student nurses are now returning to the use of a log of practical skills as a method of ensuring that they are competent and confident upon registration.

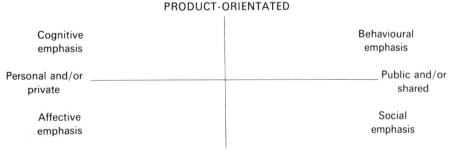

Figure 1.5 Alternative methods of teaching (Beattie 1986).

In most clinical areas, there are objectives for student placements. Students in some placements are required to make sense of the experience and link it to the theoretical underpinnings taught in college; in others, they will give hands-on care, especially during periods of rostered service. While it may be appropriate for all students to achieve the same outcomes, some students may wish to explore issues further. For example, it may be a core objective that a student is able to assess the need for analgesia for a patient in pain. To achieve this, the student needs to understand the effects of prescribed analgesics and to perceive a patient's needs accurately, while understanding the physiology and psychology associated with the experience of pain. If a learner achieves this objective, she has achieved a great deal. However, she may still be curious about pain relief and may wish you to guide her studies further.

Similarly, you may need to consider the essential knowledge, skills, insights and personal learning that your client needs to adopt in order to make a healthy recovery. Remember, however, that some clients or carers may be motivated to learn more than you initially plan so you will, therefore, have to adapt your teaching to meet their needs.

A common core curriculum (Lawton, 1987) can work well, with all students working to achieve the same objectives at the same level. However, as discussed, some students may be satisfied with what they have gained in one area but may wish for more depth in another. Lawton offers a curriculum that lends itself beautifully to adoption in the practice setting (Fig. 1.6). On the matrix, the horizontal line labelled A–D represents the core objectives that you wish each student to achieve during her allocation to your area, or that a patient/client needs to achieve in order to adapt to his condition. These core topics may be linked to the practice competencies and embrace the knowledge, skills issues and personal developments that you hope all students will gain.

The vertical line in Figure 1.6 represents additional objectives at a variety of levels and difficulties, which cater for the differing interests and abilities of the student group. For example, we have already discussed the core objective of assessing the need for analgesia for a postoperative patient or client. A student may wish to explore the place of alternative therapies, such as massage, or to consider how psychological interventions can help to alter perceptions of pain. To facilitate this, you may need to devise some guided study or a visit to a specialist nurse with a worksheet to complete.

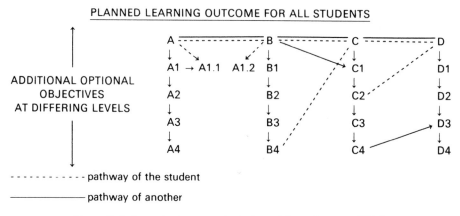

Figure 1.6 A curriculum matrix (adapted from Lawton 1975).

Lawton suggests that, for every core objective, the teacher should work out additional themes at a variety of levels and difficulty, which cater for the differing interests and abilities of the student group. Some students will spend large periods of time and require skilled facilitation to achieve a core objective, while others ascend the ladder to gain higher levels of knowledge. The student who found difficulty in one area often seeks more information and discovery in another. In this way, the richness of the clinical learning environment can be capitalised upon in a multitude of ways.

The drawback of such a model is the amount of detailed planning that is needed if the programme is to be successful. Each activity needs to be prepared so that the student is guided appropriately. Additionally, you may wish to structure activities so that as students move across and through the matrix, gaining breadth and depth, they move towards a student-centred approach. Strategies that you could prepare might include worksheets and diagrams, guided reading or visits (with guidance) to a medical museum, pathology laboratory or scanning department. You may set projects; you may develop themes that focus on activities of living, or themes that underpin the particular framework for practice that is in use. Additionally, assessment, planning, implementation and evaluation may help to determine levels, especially when linked to Benner's (1984) stages of practitioner competence.

A group of you in your practice setting could get together to develop this idea. You should find that you can build on the learning opportunities that you have to offer.

CONCLUSION

This chapter has considered the nature of teaching and the characteristics of effective and ineffective teachers. An overview of four approaches to teaching and learning has been presented, providing you with an opportunity to develop your ideas for teaching in each section. A way of structuring your teaching programme is suggested, followed by a brief consideration of factors that detract from learning.

The final task is to consider how you might develop your repertoire of teaching activities. Part of the answer lies in having a go, but understanding the knowledge base that informs teaching, practising and developing your skills, and reflecting on the practice of good role models, will all raise your awareness of issues that impinge on your teaching role and will result in your enhanced performance. You might apply the fourfold approach to yourself, by developing knowledge and skills, and by sharing teaching and learning with your peer group, reflecting with them, privately and perhaps also with a mentor. It may help if you draw up a fourfold diagram that identifies the overall approach, and as you develop in confidence, you may be able to list the skills and resources needed for each type.

GLOSSARY

Behaviourism: the study of psychology by considering an individual's behaviour rather than the functioning of the brain and nervous system.

Brainstorm: an intensive situation in which spontaneous suggestions for solutions to problems are generated by a group, without evaluation. The group later evaluates the suggestions and decides on the best alternative(s).

Cognitive learning: considers that mental processes and representations are essential to learning, so that we are not passive receptors of information but actively process incoming data, transforming it into categories and new forms.

Cognitive school of psychology: an approach to psychology that stresses the role of mental processes in understanding behaviour.

Computer-assisted learning (CAL): uses the principle of operant conditioning, in which the student's correct response is rewarded with praise and encouragement via the computer software.

Critical incident analysis: analysis of a snapshot, a moment in time when an occurrence in the daily work of the carer will affect client care. Events may be large, small, positive or negative, for example, a positive interaction between a client and carer. Learning is gained from reflection on the incident in clinical supervision or in using a structured model of reflection.

Curriculum: the education programme of an institution, which includes philosophy, teaching method and its implementation and effects.

Exposition: a period of teacher talk in which knowledge is imparted or explanations are given.

Gestalt school of psychology: a psychological theory primarily concerned with perception, which emphasises pattern organisation.

Group norms: members of a group act and expect each other to act in a particular way, for example, in terms of styles of dress or ways of interacting.

Humanistic: emphasises the qualities that distinguish people from animals. This school considers a principal motivating force to be a tendency towards growth and self-actualisation.

Perception: how we come to know what is going on around us by interpreting what is happening in ourselves and our surroundings, using senses, expectations and experience.

Process recordings: a verbatim, serial account of an interaction between two individuals.

Psychomotor skills: learning skills and procedures, coordinating sensory stimuli to achieve purposeful movement.

Rehearsal: repetition of an item or aspect of behaviour, which can transfer it into long-term memory.

Reinforcement: reinforcing a response by the presentation of a stimulus that increases the strength of the conditioning; typically, in operant conditioning, it is in the form of a reward.

Role play: students act out specific social roles for the purpose of increasing insight.

Skills analysis: breaking down a skill into small steps so that it reads like a recipe, each step forming a stimulus–response association.

Stimulus-response theory: a view that all behaviour is in response to stimuli, for example, our response to the sound of an alarm.

Syndicates: where students are divided into groups to work on the same or related problems with teacher contact as needed. The syndicate present a joint report for the whole group.

REFERENCES

Alulinas W (1978) Some case studies of unsuccessful student teachers: their implications for teacher education changes. *Teacher Educator*, **13**(3), 30–37.

Atkinson RL, Atkinson RC, Smith E, Ben D and Nolen-Hoeksema P (1996) *Introduction to Psychology*, 12th edn. New York: Harcourt Brace Jovanovich.

Bandura A (1977) *Social Learning Theory*. New Jersey: Prentice Hall.

Barton-Wright P (1994) Clinical supervision and nursing. *British Journal of Nursing*, **13**(1), 23–30.

Beattie A (1986) *Curriculum Development for Health Studies: A Foundation for Nurse Teachers. Blueprint for the Future*. London: King's Fund Centre.

Beattie A (1987) Making a curriculum work. In *The Curriculum in Nursing Education*, eds, Allan P and Jolley M. London: Croom Helm.

Benner P (1984) *From Novice to Expert*. Menlo Park CA: Addison Wesley.

Benor D and Leviyof I (1997) The development of student's perceptions of effective teaching: the ideal, best and poorest clinical teacher in nursing. *Journal of Nursing Education*, **36**(5), 206–211.

Biggs J and Moore P (1993) *The Process of Learning*. London: Prentice Hall.

Boud D, Keogh R and Walker D (1985) *Reflection: Turning Experience into Learning*. London: Kogan Page.

Burns R (1982) *Self-concept Development and Education*. London: Holt, Rinehart & Winston.

Butterworth T and Faugier J (1992) *Clinical Supervision and Mentorship in Nursing*. London: Chapman & Hall.

Child D (1997) *Psychology and the Teacher*, 5th edn. London: Holt, Rinehart & Winston.

Combs AW (1965) *The Professional Education of Teachers*, Boston, MA: Allyn & Bacon.

Cybert RM (1980) Problem-solving and education policy. In *Problem Solving and Education: Issues in Teaching and Research*, eds, Turna D and Relf F. New Jersey: Laurence Erlbaum Associates.

Davies S (1996) How can nurse teachers be more effective in practice settings? *Nurse Education Today*, **16**(1), 19–27.

Editorial (1997) *Evidence-Based Nursing*, **1**(1), 7–8.

Edwards R (1997) *Changing Places? Flexibility, Lifelong Learning and a Learning Society*. London: Routledge.

Fontana D (1972) What do we mean by a good teacher? In *Research Forum on Teacher Education*, ed. Chanan D. Windsor: National Foundation for Educational Research.

Fox DJ (1975) *Fundamentals of Research in Nursing*, 4th edn. New York: Appleton-Century-Crofts.

Fretwell J (1985) *Freedom to Change: The Creation of the Ward Learning Environment*. London: RCN.

Gage NL (1978) *The Scientific Basis of the Art of Teaching*. New York: Teachers College Press.

Henry J (1981) Evaluation of teaching skills. *South Pacific Journal of Teacher Education*, **9**(1), 61–65.

Howie J (1988) The effective clinical teacher: a role model. *Australian Journal of Advanced Nursing*, **5**(2), 23–26.

Joyce B and Weil M (1986) *Models of Teaching*, 3rd edn. London: Prentice Hall.

Lawton D (1975) *Class Culture and the Curriculum*. London: Routledge & Kegan Paul.

Lawton D (1987) The changing role of the teacher: consequences for teacher education and training. *Prospects*, **17**(1), 91–98.

Li M (1997) Perceptions of effective clinical teaching behaviours in a hospital-based nurse teaching programme. *Journal of Advanced Nursing*, **26**(6), 1252–1261.

Marson SN (1982) Ward sister–teacher or facilitator? An investigation into the behavioural characteristics of effective ward teachers. *Journal of Advanced Nursing*, **7**, 347–357.

Melia K (1983) Students' views of nursing. 4: Doing nursing and being professional. *Nursing Times*, **79**(22), 28–30.

Miles R (1987) Experiential learning in the curriculum. In *The Curriculum in Nursing Education*, eds, Allan P and Jolley M. London: Croom Helm.

Morgan J and Knox JE (1987) Characteristics and 'best' and 'worst' clinical teachers as perceived by university nursing faculty and students. *Journal of Advanced Nursing*, **12**, 331–337.

Myles A (1987) Psychology and the curriculum. In *The Curriculum in Nursing Education*, eds, Allan P and Jolley M London: Croom Helm.

Myles A (1993) Psychology and health care. In *Nursing Practice and Health Care*, 2nd edn eds, Hinchliff SM, Norman S and Schober J. London: Edward Arnold.

National Committee of Inquiry into Higher

Education (1997) *Higher Education in the Learning Society* (Dearing Reports). London: NCIHE.

Ornstein AC (1990) *Strategies for Effective Teaching*. New York: Harper & Row.

Peters RS (1977) *Education and the Education of Teachers*. London: Routledge & Kegan Paul.

Quinn FM (1995) *The Principle and Practice of Nurse Education*, 3rd edn. London: Croom Helm.

Rich A and Parker DL (1995) Reflection and critical incident analysis: ethical and moral implications of their use within nursing and midwifery education. *Journal of Advanced Nursing*, **22**, 1050–1057.

Rickman LW and Hollowell J (1981) Some causes of student teacher failure. *Improving College and University Teaching*, **29**(4), 176–178.

Rogers C (1983) *Freedom to Learn for the 80's*. Columbus, OH: Charles E., Merrill

Schön DA (1987) *Educating the Reflective Practitioner*. San Francisco: Jossey Bass.

Schonell FJ (1961) *University Teaching in Queensland*, Report of a conference for demonstrators and lecturers. Brisbane: University of Queensland Press.

Sheahan J (1980) Some aspects of the teaching and learning of nursing. *Journal of Advanced Nursing*, **5**, 491–511.

Sheffield EF (ed) (1974) *Teaching in the Universities: No One Way*. Montreal: McGill University Press.

Sherman B and Blackburn RT (1974) *Eric Abstracts*, **9**(8), 88.

United Kingdom Central Council for Nursing, Midwifery and Health Visiting (1997a) *PREP and You*. London: UKCC.

United Kingdom Central Council for Nursing, Midwifery and Health Visiting (1997b) *Standards for the Preparation of Teachers of Nursing, Midwifery and Health Visiting*. CC/97/21. London: UKCC.

Wong S (1978) Nurse-teachers' behaviours in the clinical field: apparent effect on nursing students learning. *Journal of Advanced Nursing*, **3**, 369–372.

Wragg EC (1974) *Teaching Teaching*. London: David & Charles.

Wragg EC (ed.) (1984) *Classroom Teaching Skills*. London: Croom Helm.

FURTHER READING

Atkinson RL, Atkinson RC, Smith E, Ben D and Noten-Hoeksena P et al (1996) *Introduction to Psychology*, 12th edn. New York: Harcourt Brace Jovanovich. *Useful for revising or finding out about psychological principles.*

Barton-Wright P (1994) Clinical supervision and primary nursing. *British Journal of Nursing*, **3**(1), 23–30. *Makes a positive analysis of supervision and applies it to the role of the primary nurse.*

Benner P (1984) *From Novice to Expert*. Menlo Park Cal: Addison Wesley. *The research findings and use of the Dreyfus model of skill acquisition are essential reading and will help you better to understand your students. A valuable resource.*

Benor D and Leviyof I (1997) The development of student's perceptions of effective teaching: the ideal best and poorest clinical teacher in nursing. *Journal of Nursing Education*, **36**(5), 206–211. *Useful for a contemporary comparison of an international perspective, but the principles will not surprise you.*

Biggs J and Moore P (1993) *The Process of Learning*. London: Prentice Hall. *For an interesting application and adaptation of Piaget's stages of concept formation and also for application of psychology and sociology to the process of learning.*

Bolt E (1991) *Becoming Reflective*. London: Distance Learning Centre, South Bank Polytechnic. *An imaginative distance learning pack, which allows you to explore what it is to reflect in and on your practice.*

Butterworth T and Faugier J (1992) *Clinical Supervision and Mentoring in Nursing*. London: Chapman & Hall. *An edited book that builds on the foundations of the subject and makes application to the families of nursing as well as considering the development of self. An excellent and relevant read.*

Child D (1997) *Psychology and the Teacher*, 5th edn. London: Holt, Reinehart and Winston. *An easy-to-read introduction to educational psychology.*

Davies S (1996) How can nurse teachers be more effective in practice settings? *Nurse Education Today*, **16**(1), 19–27. *The title really says it all; useful to consolidate the discussion in the chapter.*

Evidence Based Nursing vol. 1, no 1, particularly the Editorial 'Closing the gap between research and practice' on pages 7 and 8. *Additionally, the journal is a formative read as a source of research for practice.*

Fretwell J (1985) *Freedom to Change: The Creation of the Ward Learning Environment*. London: RCN. *Essential reading about the role of the ward sister.*

Hargie O (ed.) (1986) *A Handbook of Communication Skills*. London: Croom Helm. *Provides an interesting and readable theoretical account of communication.*

Heum C (1980) *Communication in Nursing Practice*, 2nd edn. Boston: Little, Brown. *This considers and applies communication skills to nursing.*

Johnson W (1990) *Reaching Out*, 4th edn. London: Prentice Hall. *The book offers practical exercises that can help you develop your skills in communicating.*

Li M 1997 Perceptions of effective clinical teaching behaviours in a hospital based teaching programme. *Journal of Advanced Nursing*, **26**(6), 1252–1261. *Useful for an international perspective and to compare this with the UK.*

Marson SN (1982) Ward sister – teacher or facilitator? An investigation into the behavioural characteristics of effective ward teachers. *Journal of Advanced Nursing*, **7**, 347–357.

Rich A and Parker DL (1995) Reflection and critical incident analysis: ethical and moral implications of their use within nursing and midwifery education. *Journal of Advanced Nursing*, **22**, 1050–1057. *This article clearly details factors that must be taken into account when using models of reflection as a teaching tool.*

Rogers C (1983) *Freedom to Learn for the 80's*. Columbus, Ohio: Charles E. Meril. *Rogers describes one way of facilitating student-centred learning and the background philosophy. This book, although now quite old, is an absolute classic, particularly the earlier chapters where Rogers describes his own journey in teaching.*

United Kingdom Central Council for Nursing, Midwifery and Health Visiting (1997) *PREP and You*. London: UKCC.

United Kingdom Central Council for Nursing, Midwifery and Health Visiting (1997) *Standards for the Preparation of Teachers of Nursing, Midwifery and Health Visiting*. CC/97/21. *Useful for definitions of the term 'mentor' and its application to the role of the teacher. Also a positive example of the style of paper that the statutory body presents to its Council.*

2 The world in which learning and teaching take place

Sally Thomson

INTRODUCTION

The education of adults takes place under two main umbrellas. The first is higher education, which includes all the universities in the UK. The **university** function will be explored in detail as the focal point of this chapter. The second umbrella is further education. Many of you will have participated in further education evening classes or worked with colleagues undertaking **National Vocational Qualifications** or those who have undertaken specific training at one of these colleges. The divide is crude as there are often overlapping activities between further and higher education, but on the whole, they are funded and function differently. 'A' level qualifications offer a common point for the differences, with universities tending to work *above* this standard and further education colleges tending to offer courses *up* to this level. It is higher education that has the most relevance for preregistration nursing education at present.

This chapter aims to help you to understand the world of higher education. Some of you will read it from start to finish; many of you will dip in and out of it as need dictates. Both approaches are acceptable, although there are some useful activities in this section that may help you with your own profile development.

The glossary will also help as a quick reference point. There are not many reflective points or activities in this chapter as it is intended as an underpinning and support to the rest of the book.

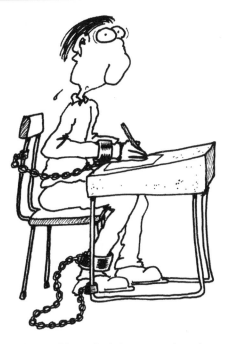

The world in which learning takes place

LEARNING OBJECTIVES

After reading this chapter, you should be able to:

- describe the structure and function of a university
- explain the funding mechanisms for higher education
- outline the higher education quality mechanisms
- understand the student lifestyle and financial support mechanisms
- be able to locate your own study pathway within an academic arena.

THE HIGHER EDUCATION SYSTEM

ACTIVITY 2.1

Jot down some ideas about what you think the role of a **university** might be.

Many of you will have thought of the main function of a university as offering knowledge or learning. Bligh (1990) makes the point that higher education is a national resource for knowledge, but not exclusively so, as databases, museums and libraries are also sources of knowledge, so learning is not exclusively the remit of the higher education system.

You may have considered the preparation of nurses as a function of the university sector, and if you broaden the principles of this, it becomes apparent that the nation's economy is tied into the development of a skilled workforce. Additionally, education is designed to develop an individual's intellect and ability; another core function of a university is to develop knowledge through research, which will, in turn, advance learning.

Finally, the Robbins Committee (DoE, 1963) considered one of the aims of education to be the transmission of a common culture. This latter aim is complex and intended to be interpreted liberally. It is concerned with handing on values, standards of citizenship, social skills and the preservation of a democracy. The Dearing Report (DfEE, 1997) recommends that higher education creates a learning society, with lifelong learning as the key to responding to change – personal, professional and societal.

If you refer back to Chapter 1, you will see the ideals of education translated into the fourfold curriculum model in Figure 1.1. The section on learning as a cultural activity is an exercise laden with such values.

The Dearing Report on higher education

In 1996, Sir Ron Dearing (now Lord Dearing) was commissioned by all the political parties to conduct a major review of higher education. The report is in many sections, the main document referring to England, Wales and Northern Ireland. The second section of the report is known as the Garrick Report and is concerned with Scotland, aiming to preserve the uniqueness of the Scottish system while ensuring that the quality approach that underpins the whole Report is integrated into Scotland. The Report was published in the summer of 1997 with 93 recommendations relevant to the next 10 years. The basic underpinning of the review is that people from all walks of life will continue in education and training in order to keep pace with rapid change in the world, at work and in their lives. The Report states that its aim is to 'encourage and enable all students … whether they demonstrate the highest intellectual potential or whether they have struggled to reach the threshold of higher education'. The report claims that higher education will:

- enable economic competitiveness
- support the richness of our culture
- foster the values of a cohesive, democratic and pluralist society.

You might like to refer back to your response to Activity 2.1 and compare it with the Dearing recommendations.

A huge consultation exercise resulted from this, and in 1998 the Department for Education and Employment issued a Green Consultation Paper on lifelong learning, entitled *The Learning Age*, which responds to the report *Higher Education in the Learning Society* and its resultant feedback. The Dearing Report is optimistic in nature: it describes how universities, with their research base, can support a knowledge-based economy, encouraging motivation and innovation that enables society to understand and adapt to change. Three core intentions are expressed in the report (Box 2.1).

BOX 2.1	*Proposals of the Dearing Report (DfEE, 1997)*

1. Access to higher education is to be increased. Wider participation is to be encouraged by students from underrepresented groups, such as ethnic minorities and those with disabilities.
2. Education must be of a high quality, which is to be supported by a new Institute for Learning and Teaching in higher education.
3. Standards are to be guaranteed, supported by a code of practice and a new framework of qualifications that integrates National Vocational Qualifications with the traditional academic pathway.

Many of the recommendations from the Report will be mentioned as the chapter progresses, but its summary and recommendations are well worth reading.

THE UNIVERSITY

It quickly becomes apparent that a university's core function is to develop knowledge through research and then to transmit this by creating a complementary teaching and learning environment.

Education, however, is a national resource and, as such, receives its finance and support from government, through the Department for Education and Employment. In turn, the accountability process goes upwards from the university to government. Teaching and research are supported through a dual funding system. Bligh (1990) indicates that universities were established by a Royal Charter, and this prevents interference by government in what is taught and researched. This academic freedom is not universal in other countries.

From the first exercise you may also have noted that universities design, **validate** and administer their own courses. They deal with student assessment and grant their own awards. Universities each have their own colours and corporate design that adorn the traditional academic dress of a graduate.

Universities are often identified by whether they are an ancient university, red-brick or new. Two examples of ancient universities are Oxford and Cambridge, which were founded in the Middle Ages and have many different colleges forming each university. These universities have their own entrance requirements. Such universities tend to dominate a city, the colleges often being built around a courtyard and each with its own chapel. The system of learning rests on the tutorial (a small group of students or a one-to-one system in which an academic challenge is explored and personal work monitored), and prestigious scholarships are often offered for entrants. Historically, the old universities were renowned for their research.

A red-brick university is the label attached to the old civic universities that sprang up to serve the adult local community, teaching by a central method (the traditional pattern of learning in the lecture room). These institutions were encouraged to provide vocational courses which were often run part time. They were frequently characterised by links developed with industry. Manchester and

Durham are examples of this group. Even today, they retain their local interests, for example, textiles at Leeds and music at Manchester, but they tend to have a broad academic base that has developed to make provision for local need. However, Palfreyman and Warner (1996) caution against increasing confusion in the labelling of universities by trying to simplify the titles.

Newer civic universities used to provide courses validated by London University; Southampton is an example of this. The system required the university to match the standard of London University in a kind of apprenticeship before being able to confer its own degrees and awards. After the Second World War, new universities emerged that tended to have a specialist function as a result of the award of large amounts of research funding; one example is that of sociology at Essex. In addition, at this time, colleges of advanced technology were awarded university status. Finally, in the 1980s, 29 polytechnics were awarded university status, forming what are called the 'new universities'. Although the term 'old' and 'red-brick' remain, many universities have amalgamated and merged as part of the ongoing developments and changes in education.

The 'virtual' university is now offering courses to students. Thames Valley University offers a programme that is accessed from home using the Internet. In addition, programmes ranging from certificate to degree are available through universities that use distance learning as the medium for teaching and learning; the Open University is a key example of this.

The governance of universities

Universities are self-governing, the responsibility for them resting with the Secretary of State for Education and Employment in England and the Secretaries of State in Scotland, Wales and Northern Ireland. Advice to the government on matters related to universities is provided by the Higher Education Funding Councils for England, Wales and Scotland, and by the Northern Ireland Higher Education Council (*Whitaker's Almanack*, 1997).

Every university, prior to the integration of polytechnics into universities, had a **chancellor** as its titular head. This is an honorary and ceremonial appointment, and the chancellor usually presides at meetings of the university's governing body and at award-giving ceremonies. The **vice-chancellor** is the chief academic and administrative officer and is responsible for the day-to-day running of the university. The **registrar** is in charge of administration. Edwards (1994) describes the changing role of the vice-chancellor, who has to protect the fundamental mission of the university while responding continuously to change in order to ensure the survival of the institution in a rapidly changing world. Edwards (1994) describes how the vice-chancellor must create a climate of anticipation in order to keep pace with rapid change.

The university structure

A university structure is mapped out in Figure 2.1. the basic building blocks of the structure are the departments and at the top of the hierarchy is the **senate**.

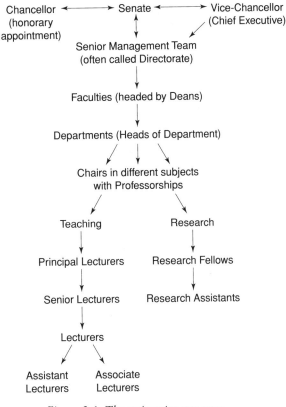

Figure 2.1 The university structure.

The department

The basic unit of university organisation is the department, defined by subject specialism. This is where most lecturers feel they belong. Many of you will be studying in, and affiliated to, a health studies or midwifery or nursing department, or one named with a combination of these terms.

Traditionally, a **head of department** leads this basic unit, and tends to be the focus of communications and decisions. The head is also the person who usually represents the department in the broader university machinery. The head may or may not be a professor and may have competed for the post or been elected by peers. Members of the department will also have different status, ranging from **professor** to **reader** to senior lecturer to **lecturer** and sometimes even to assistant, associate or visiting lecturer.

Faculties/schools

Faculties or **schools** are groups of affiliated subject departments. For example, the social sciences may be grouped together, and in some universities, nursing and medical studies combine to form a faculty. Most students will study under the umbrella of a single faculty. Faculties strive for common standards in such areas as course assessment and programme validation, and comparison between departments is a key feature of a faculty. Rules and regulations are part of a faculty's way of being. The faculty is regulated by a **dean** who manages processes through a faculty board. Again, the dean may have been elected by peers or have applied for the position. The dean may or may not be a senior professor.

The faculty is monitored by a faculty board, which exercises quality control and is concerned with standards, also acting as an intermediary for the complex communications that need to take place within a university. The faculty board has a formal process, operating through a traditional committee mechanism of agenda and reports.

ACTIVITY 2.2

Attend a faculty board as observer or, if this is difficult, read the minutes, which will be in the library. Either will give you an overview of a faculty's life and work. Plot from the agenda and minutes the make-up of the board, the number of different titles and the complexity of communications that go on between departments.

You will see from this that people are often affiliated to more than one department and are engaged in a variety of activities. Collections of individuals may work together to validate a course, conduct research or teach a module in what seems to be a chaotic way, but this is perhaps best understood from the principles of project management, in which groups of people come together to perform a specific function but may not relate to each other in a direct organisational line. Most people in a university will function within several functional project groups at one time.

Senate

The senate is the senior academic committee of the university. Usually, the heads of all the academic departments sit on the senate. University regulations also require the presence of lay members. The senate is chaired by the university's most senior academic: the vice-chancellor, **director** or **principal**, depending on the terminology and infrastructure in use.

The senate is the supreme governing body (Bligh, 1990). It stipulates academic policies and procedures, and is the final level of appeal on academic matters. The senate usually has a web of subcommittees to support its work.

University governance

University governance is directed from a council or **board of governors**. Up to half of the committee will consist of lay members. These will come from the local education authority, business or industry, and the board will also contain some distinguished members from other walks of life who take part in university governance. The university representatives will represent the senate, faculties, students and junior lecturers as part of its democratic process. Board business includes staff appointments and promotions, allocating resources, overseeing the budget and bidding for finance from external sources. Council appoints the members of the senate. Joint committees of senate and council are becoming increasingly common. Dearing (DfEE, 1997) suggests that governors review their objectives, on a 5-yearly cycle, to evaluate the effectiveness of the university and their leadership. Universities may devise their own indicators of success but must also monitor themselves against new, nationally agreed standards. Part of this analysis will be the handling of complaints.

Support structures

Although the university is academic in nature, it could not function without a host of support services, including the library, the **registry**, the management of information systems, public relations, porters, accommodation staff and estate managers. Each institution will have a professional administration responsible for all non-academic activities, including accounting, upkeep of the buildings and capital investment.

THE FUNDING OF HIGHER EDUCATION

There are two main sources of funding for higher education: the first supports teaching and learning activities, and the second resources research activity. The funding of higher education is represented in Figure 2.2.

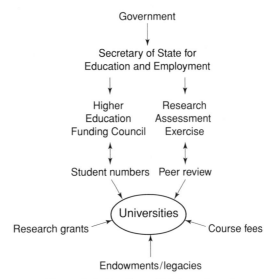

Figure 2.2 Funding of higher education.

The Higher Education Funding Council (HEFC) for each country makes an annual grant to each institution for the coming academic year (August to July). The exception is Northern Ireland, where the grant is allocated centrally from government. The money is primarily to support teaching, but it also includes some funding for research. In order to realise the money, the institution is required to maintain a specific number of student enrollments, the formula being designed to promote efficiency and stability. In essence, the money is given to contract specific student numbers from the UK and the European Union. Failure to reach enrollment targets results in the HEFC clawing back some of its monies.

Extra funds may also be allocated from HEFC on a competitive basis. The funding councils exist, *inter alia*, to monitor the financial health of a university; that is, they are concerned with good management practice and value for money.

HEFC money is controlled by the Secretary of State for Education by direct grant from the government. Members of HEFCs are appointed by government and are drawn from universities, industry and commerce.

Research funds are allocated using a different system to meet direct project costs. The research assessment exercise (RAE) is a competitive exercise, managed using peer review. Institutions that enter the assessment receive a rating from 1 to 5, 5 being the highest score. A high rating in the RAE carries enormous kudos. Dearing (1997) proposed that the RAE be redesigned to end the competitive process and to encourage partnerships and collaboration in research. This would allow universities to learn from and adopt each other's good practice, and allow initiatives to be shared. Dearing also called for increased funding for research activity and for research projects to be shared with industry. Finally, Dearing recommends the formation of an Arts and Humanities Council, which would give support and status to the qualitative methods of research that are so essential to making sense of nursing.

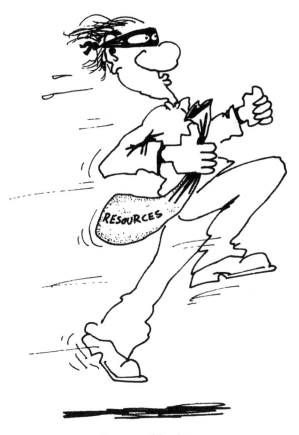

Sources of funding

Universities are multimillion pound businesses, other sources of income including HEFC capital grants for building maintenance and so on, endowments and legacies, research grants and contracts from one of the six research councils. Income is generated from consultancy as well as from course fees that are levied by each institution at a level agreed by the senate.

THE QUALITY OF EDUCATION

Funding councils also have a statutory duty to assess the quality of education provision of universities and colleges. The body responsible for this role is the Quality Assurance Agency for Higher Education (QAAHE). The agency has a core of permanent staff but also recruits subject specialists from the university sector who work within a system of peer review, that is, a review of an institution's work by a team of assessors, who are lecturers in the same subject from another university, visit an institution over a period of days and rate the quality of the provision by sitting in on taught sessions with the students, listening and questioning students and lecturers, reviewing evaluation data and gathering evidence from a broad repertoire of documentation. The reports are available to the public.

Assessment takes place cyclically, determined by subject. Nursing is due for review at the time of writing, but the changes in the funding of preregistration courses in 1997 means that it is in fact unlikely to be reviewed at this point (see Chapter 3).

Educational quality is also monitored in-house by rigorous university mechanisms. The proposal to run a course is scrutinised in a formal meeting of a validation panel managed by the university as part of a process of quality assurance and improvement. Members of the panel will include subject experts from outside the institution, members of a different internal faculty, the lecturers and dean who propose to run the course, and prospective and past students. In nursing courses that are approved by one of the National Boards, representatives from the board will also be present, it then being termed 'conjoint' validation. The course document is a detailed proposal, ranging from the philosophy of the programme to detailed indicative reading lists that are subject to scrutiny. As a result of this, approval is given or withheld, and conditions and recommendations are made about the future running of the course.

Dearing (DfEE, 1997) sees the standard and quality of education as key issues. Part of upholding standards will be achieved by strengthening the external examiner system to create a UK-wide pool. The report sees a national credit transfer scheme and the adoption of a national awards framework as a crucial step in this process.

THE ACADEMIC STAFF

Each university will appoint its own academic staff, adopting its own terms and conditions of work. There is, however, a common salary structure and a similar career pattern. The academic pathway begins at the level of assistant and associate lecturer; lecturers move on to senior lecturer and then progresses to principal lecturer and head of department. The academic research pathway begins at the level of researcher and moves on through **fellow** and reader to professor. A professor may hold a '**chair**'. Chairs can be 'personal', that is, they are awarded for personal contributions of significant merit, or positional, in which, for example, the senior academic nursing position in a university holds a chair or the title of professor. Such chairs can be applied for, whereas personal chairs are conferred. Traditionally, promotion relies on an extensive research profile.

Lecturing staff in higher education require no formal teaching qualification at present. However, the Dearing Report recommends that all teachers in higher education should be able to demonstrate teaching skills; these can be achieved either by a formal programme, in-house training or accreditation.

In 1997, a survey was carried out exploring the role of the lecturer (National Association for Teachers in Further and Higher Education (NATFHE), 1997). Overall, there was a male: female ratio of 2:1; nearly half of the sample were aged between 45 and 54; 93% of the staff were on full-time contracts; 47% lectured for 15 hours or more per week; 43% spent 15 hours or more per week preparing for sessions; and, in addition, 35% had lectured for 25 or more hours per week. The latter finding goes against a national agreement that formal scheduled teaching should not exceed more than 18 hours a week. The biggest increase in the lecturer's work was reported as being in administration. A third of lecturers reported taking half or less of their holiday, and 98% took work home at weekends. Nearly half of the sample were involved in the RAE and felt pressured to contribute to this. Thirty-nine per cent felt that lecturing detracted from their research time. It is evident that the amount of preparatory work needed to conduct a lesson contributes significantly to a lecturer's workload. The lecturer's age profile may indicate that many lecturers are appointed after a successful career and may maximise on that experience as a platform for teaching.

THE STUDENTS

The target number for students set by government is 35% of the 18–19-year-old age group by 2002. Quotas are set for medical, dental and veterinary students, but there are no limits set for other subjects (*Whitaker's Almanack*, 1997). The formal entry requirements for most degree programmes is two 'A' levels at grade E or above, and most universities set their own entrance ceiling that is above this.

Students currently apply for a course through a central clearing house called the Universities and Colleges Admission Service (UCAS). UCAS supplies a handbook and application forms, and these are readily available from schools and colleges as well as directly from UCAS. Applicants may apply for eight courses on the form. UCAS operates a strict equal opportunities policy. The Open University is the exception to this process, running its own admission service.

UCAS applications are submitted between September and December each year. In August – September of the following year, it operates a clearing house system, matching vacancies to unplaced students.

Student life may focus around where the students live, either in halls of residence or in flats and hostels. Outside formal learning activities, students organise clubs and societies, focusing on anything from sports to politics, and many students traditionally have access to a debating forum. The amount of time the student spends in taught sessions on a full-time course is usually around 20 hours per week, and many take time to adjust to the use of free time and self-directed study. Universities usually have a chaplain, a health centre, a careers service, restaurants, welfare and counselling services, libraries and study support, including support with information technology.

Every university has a student union (usually part of the National Union of Students, or NUS), which organises social events, usually has a bar and a shop and offers a large degree of student support. In addition, the student union represents students' interests on the various university committees.

THE COURSES

Course provision is offered through full-time and part-time attendance. This can be delivered through day-release, sandwich or block-release course. Traditionally, the academic year begins in September, but the introduction of modules, units of learning and semesters (a block of learning spaced through a number of weeks rather than programmed through the year) has broken down the traditional pattern of terms, and many universities have an intake two or three times a year. Dearing (DfEE, 1997) recommends that students receive a programme that has core outcomes specifying the skills to be learned, that within course work experience is maximised upon through placements that apply learning to the world of work, and that partnerships are formed between universities and business in order to offer work experience as part of the course.

Dearing (DfEE, 1997) recommends a learning and teaching environment that is responsive to students' needs. Central to this vision is the establishment of an Institute for Learning and Teaching, which will have a key role in enhancing the value placed on teaching as an activity. The institute could also play an important part in developing national standards for the accreditation of teaching in institutions (Committee of Vice-Chancellors and Principals (CVCP), 1997).

A credit accumulation and transfer scheme (CATS) is a system of placing credit upon study that is widely recognised (Figure 2.3). It allows a student to achieve a final qualification or award by accumulating credits for the different courses of study that are successfully undertaken, and, may credit periods of professional experience. This is often called assessment of prior learning (APL) or assessment of prior experiential learning (APEL). In England, Wales and Northern Ireland, higher education courses begin with credit points offered at academic level 1 which is equivalent to certificate level; level 2 study equates with a diploma, and level 3 study is pitched at degree level. In Scotland, SCOTCATS are used, and the levels are different, reflecting the difference between Scottish Highers and the 'A' levels that are studied in the remainder of the UK.

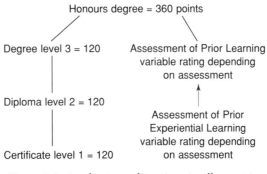

Figure 2.3 Academic credit ratings in all countries of the UK except Scotland.

Most courses with the award of degree are run over 3 years or occasionally 4, with the exception of Scotland, where traditionally, a Bachelor's degree takes 4 years. However, if students are transferring credits already accumulated towards a degree, periods of study will vary in length. Figure 2.3 maps out the credit pathway.

At postgraduate level (that is, after a Bachelor's or first degree), courses begin with Master's level, with postgraduate certificates and diplomas counting towards a Master's award. This is followed by Master of Philosophy (MPhil) and finally Doctor of Philosophy (DPhil at some universities and PhD at others), both of which are research degrees.

Once the title of Doctor of Philosophy has been achieved, there are opportunities for postdoctoral research.

ACTIVITY 2.3

From the portfolio of lifelong learning that you completed in Chapter 1, identify formal learning where you may be eligible for or have gained CATS points. Obtain a prospectus from your local university (there is usually a table of credit rating in this), and plot your credits.

Now examine what you have learned from experience; identify areas in which the learning was significant and may gain a credit rating. If you were to present this to a university for credit, you would be expected to adopt a reflective framework as outlined in Chapter 1.

You may find that your basic registration as a midwife or a nurse will give you all the points you need at level 1. This often depends on how long ago you trained. If you completed a diploma preregistration programme, you will find that you have all the points you need at level 2. It is really important that you avoid doing unnecessary study at any particular level, because if you get more points than you need at, for example, level 2, nothing will convert these to level 3 points. If you are embarking on a course of study and are beginning by selecting modules or units of learning, it is essential that you plan a learning pathway in your portfolio so that you identify what you need, work towards that and avoid unnecessary repetition.

FEES AND GRANTS

Until 1998, education was free for full-time students in the 16–19-year-old age range, although part-time students and applicants aged 19 and over were expected to pay course fees. From the 1998–99 academic year, students will be eligible to pay an annual £1000 tuition fee, with the exception of teachers, medical students, dental students and students of nursing and midwifery.

Students in the UK who undertake a full-time course of study may be eligible for a **grant**. A grant is awarded through a system of means-testing, using a sliding scale based on parental or spouse's income. If a student is 25 years or older and has been self-supporting for 3 years, a parental contribution is not deducted. It is envisaged that students will increasingly support themselves through student loans. Tuition fees are paid by students if the family income is over £35 000 per year. In Scotland, grants are awarded by the Students Award Agency, but in the other three countries of the UK, they are paid by the local education authority (LEA) and reimbursed by government. Applications are made to the authority in which the student normally lives and should be received in the January of the year of the start of the course.

Students are eligible to apply for loans through the Student Loans Company, and repayment is normally over a number of years, although this can be deferred if income is at or below a target specified by the Department for Education and Employment.

Access funds are available from the universities direct, via the faculty registry. They are available for students whose access to education may be restricted by hardship or who face financial difficulties during the course.

CONCLUSION

The mechanisms of higher education may seem complex, but the principles are the same as those operating within any national resource. Indeed, many of the codes of conduct and procedures are mirrored in the running of your local NHS Trust. Although nurse education has integrated into higher education, there are some fundamental differences, which will be dealt with in the next chapter.

GLOSSARY

Board of governors: the regulating committee of the university.

Chair: a teaching or research post of eminence. The post-holder usually has the title of professor, and the post is normally supported by an endowment.

Chancellor: the chairman of the highest decision-making body of a university. The role requires a measure of detachment from day-to-day administration, and the position is usually honorary.

Dean: a senior member of academic staff with special responsibility for discipline, pastoral care and/or administration within a faculty.

Director: the principal or head of an educational establishment.

Faculty: a division of an educational establishment made up of several departments.

Fellow: a member of the research team who contributes to teaching: sometimes a position sponsored by business or industry.

Grant: financial support for studies, paid through the local education authority.

Head of department: a member of the academic staff responsible for organising a particular academic department or teaching of a particular academic subject across the university.

Lecturer: a teacher who, by traditional title, instructs through lecture and seminar. Status can range from assistant lecturer to senior lecturer and principal lecturer.

National Vocational Qualifications: a system of awards that rest upon outcomes as a measure of the students' and course's success.

Principal: the head of an educational establishment.

Professor: the highest rank of university teacher, the title holder usually having a significant profile of major research projects.

Pro-vice-chancellor: deputy to the vice-chancellor in a university hierarchy.

Reader: the next highest rank to that of professor.

Registry: the centre for administration of university's academic performance.

Senate: the supreme academic authority of a university.

University: an institution of higher education with a strong reputation for research or teaching, or both. It is a corporate body that is able to award its own degrees.

Validation: usually carried out by a committee that is charged with assessing whether a course is able to realise what it sets out to achieve.

Vice-chancellor: the chief executive of a university.

REFERENCES

Bligh D (1990) *Higher Education*. London: Cassell.

Committee of Vice Chancellors and Principals (CVCP) (1997) *A New Partnership, Universities, Students, Business and the Nation*. London: CVCP.

Edwards K (1994) In Weil S (ed.) *Introducing Change from the Top in Universities and Colleges*. London: Kogan Page.

Department for Education and Employment (1997) *Higher Education in the Learning Society* (Dearing Report). London: HMSO.

Department for Education and Employment (1998) *The Learning Age*. London: HMSO.

National Association for Teachers in Further and Higher Education (NATFHE) (1997) *The Lecturer's Job: A Survey of Conditions of Service in the New Universities and Colleges of Higher Education*. London: NATFHE.

Palfreyman D and Warner D (eds) (1996) *Higher Education Management: The Key Elements*. Buckingham: Society for Research into Higher Education/Open University Press.

Department of Education (1963) *Higher Education*. Report of the Committee Appointed by the Prime Minister (Robbins Report) London: HMSO.

Whitaker's Almanack (1997) London: J Whitaker & Sons.

FURTHER READING

References Services, Central Office of Information (1995) *Education after 16*. London: HMSO. *One of a series of books that explains aspects of Britain, this is written in an easy style that provides a useful back-up.*

3 Nursing education is different

Sally Thomson

INTRODUCTION

This chapter builds upon the mapping of higher education that began in Chapter 2. Like the previous chapter, you may choose to read it from beginning to end or to dip into the sections according to need. However, if you are not reading sequentially, you may find that you need to cross-refer between sections, especially to the glossary of terms.

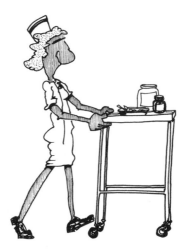

Nursing education is different

At the time of writing, nurses are educated in 89 universities in the UK. There are approximately 47 000 students studying for nursing diplomas and degrees at preregistration level, in addition to midwifery students at diploma and degree level, and a large student body working towards postgraduate qualifications. The students are taught by a workforce of 5000 nursing, midwifery and health visiting lecturers, with a core of 37 professors of nursing, most of whom are women.

You may find this chapter useful if you are considering a career pathway that embraces nurse education, but it is mainly designed to help you to function in, and develop your role as a teacher in the practice setting.

LEARNING OBJECTIVES

After reading this chapter, you should be able to:

- describe the factors that prompted the move of nurse education from NHS Trusts to higher education
- consider the lifestyle of the 'average' nursing student and reflect upon the issues that he faces
- explain the principles of commissioning and the role of education consortia
- state the differences in the two types of preregistration education
- consider your role in the reduction of the theory–practice gap and how you can develop this role
- make sense of the working life of the nurse teacher.

THE MOVE OF NURSE EDUCATION INTO HIGHER EDUCATION

Apart from a small number of university departments that were established in the 1960s to provide nursing degrees, nurse education was traditionally located at hospital sites, at the point of delivery of patient care. Many readers will have gained their initial training for caring in a school of midwifery or nursing, usually located in their hospital grounds, perhaps travelling to other units to gain specific experience. At this time, the registered nurse and midwife qualification was not located within an academic framework, and its educational currency was difficult to estimate. Values often revolved around whether or not the training took place at a teaching hospital.

In 1997, however, nurse education completed its move into higher education within the UK as the schools of nursing in Northern Ireland moved into Queen's University, Belfast. Three major events impacted upon this shift in a variety of ways:

1. In 1986, the United Kingdom Central Council for Nursing, Midwifery and Health Visiting (UKCC) (1986) published the plans for a new preparation for preregistration nurse education. Key features were a common foundation programme for all branches of nursing – adult, child health, learning disability and mental health – setting the level of the course at a diploma, with all the

academic standards that this would impose, and finally, recommending a closer collaboration between schools of nursing and the adult education sector.

2. This change was compounded by the 1990 NHS and Community Care Act, the enactment of which meant that schools of nursing no longer had a place within NHS Trusts, which lost the remit to support activity outside the sphere of care. Two things resulted from this: first, a pressure for nurse education to merge with higher education, and second, the end of each hospital recruiting the number of nursing students needed to support its own workforce, with national workforce planning taking over from the local assessment of need.

3. The abolition of the distinction between universities and polytechnics. All institutions of higher education adopted the name 'university' (Scott, 1993), and with this change of title there was, for nurse education, a massive change to its way of being.

The future of nurse education now also holds some positive challenges, not least from the Dearing Report on higher education (Department for Education and Employment, 1997) and the changes that this will effect in adult education as a whole, but also from the increasing demands for preregistration nurse education to become a graduate programme (Royal College of Nursing, 1995). The system of preregistration education is also challenged by issues to do with an ever-developing knowledge base and rapid changes of health care provision in this country.

THE COMMISSIONING OF NURSING, MIDWIFERY AND HEALTH VISITING EDUCATION

Nursing education, unlike mainstream education, exists in a purchaser/provider scenario. In higher education, the purchaser is either the Higher Education Funding Council (HEFC) or the individual student; in nursing and midwifery education, the purchaser is an education consortium and the provider is the university. The provider scenario is competitive, with the likelihood of several universities competing for the same contract. Education contracts usually run for a 5-year period, and the security of the staff and the department rests upon the contract being won. The purchaser–provider relationship for nursing and midwifery education should not be taken for granted.

In April 1996, new arrangements for the planning and commissioning of education and training in the NHS were put into place, but these excluded medical and dental education.

Education consortia, organised on a geographical basis, represent the education and workforce interests of local health care providers and purchasers. Each consortium includes representatives from the providers and purchasers of education, relevant NHS Trusts, health authorities, GPs and the local authority. Most consortia also include representatives from the non-NHS public sector and the independent and voluntary sector (Humphries, 1988). Education consortia have two main purposes:

1. to collate the workforce plans received from service providers
2. to convert the workforce plans into an 'expression' of future demand for newly qualified staff (Humphries, 1988), that is, to link service objectives to training needs (National Health Service Executive 1997a).

Humphries describes the frustration of planning and predicting 5-year work-force plans. Stock (1996) believes that many Trusts lack the historical data needed as a basis for future projections and also expresses concern at the absence of the skills needed for workforce planning. Humphries describes how workforce planning may be undermined by the absence of independent health care employers from consortia. Hence workforce plans will not be submitted from them, yet they employ professional health care staff. Finally, student nurse attrition will further complicate the workforce planning task.

Regional education development groups (REDGs) advise education consortia and maintain an overview. They examine workforce plans submitted by regionally based consortia and interpret the implications for the region as a whole, the eight REDGs then submit their plans to the National Health Service Executive (NHSE) for analysis. The NHSE explores workforce trends on a national basis and, in analysing regional plans, considers financial issues and other factors. Figure 3.1 summarises the workforce planning exercise that results in the number of student places that are purchased. The NHSE is responsible for maintaining an adequate supply of nurses and midwives for the NHS and works on a system that is 5 years ahead of need, since it has to take into account the amount of time it takes to recruit and train the workforce.

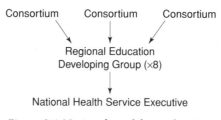

Figure 3.1 National workforce planning.

ACTIVITY 3.1

Analyse the nursing or midwifery workforce requirements for your clinical area using the off-duty rota. How can you predict the changing needs for 5 years time? What education will be needed to keep the nursing workforce skilled and ready to adapt to future needs?

You may have identified trends such as the increasing use of technology, rapid patient throughput, the increasing incidence of specific illnesses such as tuberculosis, or changes in procedures, for example, minimally invasive therapies. Next, you have to decide how many staff will need reskilling in order to keep abreast of changing trends, and how you will purchase a high-quality education programme that is effective and represents value for money. You have already begun to work and think as a purchaser of education. If you multiply this exercise by the number of clinical areas in your Trust and the number of Trusts in your region, you can begin to understand the complexity of the purchasing exercise. This is complicated by the unexpected; for example, no purchaser of education would have had a 5-year warning of the need to care for clients who are HIV positive. Added to this, with a restricted sum of money, you have to prioritise and work out a strategy to do this. From here, you can see that the purchase of health care education is a highly political issue.

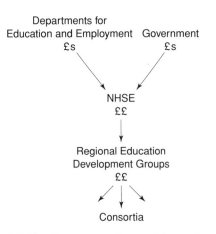

Figure 3.2 Funding sources for workforce planning.

The role of consortia

Within consortia, there are specific roles and responsibilities:

- The consortium chair is nominated by the members and approved by the regional director to represent the interests of the consortium externally. The chair will account to the REDG for the work of the group and is there to exercise a leadership role and manage the business of the group. The consortium business manager manages operational functions, putting systems and processess into place and ensuring that the business plan is delivered. This is a pivotal role.
- The consortium is not a legal entity, and Trusts and health authorities will need to employ staff whose role will be to engage with consortia duties and manage finances.
- Trusts and health authorities are responsible for the use of non-medical education and training (NMET) money (allocated by the Department of Health) and for guaranteeing that the financial systems in place represent value for money. Trusts have the workforce planning systems that provide the data that consortia need to operate. A health authority will ensure that the consortium is supplied with service planning and commissioning intentions so that it can respond with education and training intentions.
- GPs, as purchasers and providers of health care, have a key role in consortia; they also represent the education needs of all those involved in primary care.
- The social services and voluntary sectors are also providers of health care and rely on staff prepared by the NHS. They can provide valuable workforce data. The NHSE (National Health Service Executive, 1997a) stresses that their participation in the planning of the overall health care workforce is essential to matching supply and demand. In addition, this sector also commissions education and training.
- The REDG has an important advisory role in consortia.

The members of a consortium are mapped out in Figure 3.3, and its functions are summarised in Box 3.1.

BOX 3.1	*Functions of a consortium*

- To foster understanding between commissioners and higher education providers
- To provide links with medical and dental education and workforce issues
- To examine the educational implications of new policies and service developments
- To discuss educational issues across the money divide and NHS Trusts
- To support new developments in education provision in line with strategic plans
- To work on problems common to consortia and which they wish to tackle on a joint basis
- To ensure that the views of consortia within the region are represented nationally (National Health Service Executive, 1997a)

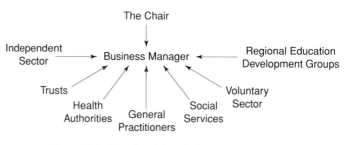

Figure 3.3 Membership of education consortia.

The NHSE charges consortia with:

1. prequalifying education and training required to gain entry into employment as a health care professional
2. a commitment to continuing education and lifelong learning for health care professionals
3. changing modes of programme delivery: modular part-time programmes, open and distance learning, and flexible courses delivered in a variety of forms
4. shared learning to support teamworking across professional and organisational boundaries
5. preparing the health care workforce to provide a coherent service within a primary care-led NHS and across health and social care boundaries
6. development priorities for employers and national priorities to meet service objectives.

The 5-yearly cycle of commissioning poses an unremitting strain upon nurse academics, who are in a constant cycle of response to commissioners' needs in order to protect the number of student places and, in turn, their own jobs.

THE FUNDING OF NURSING AND MIDWIFERY EDUCATION

In September 1998, the system for funding the preregistration education of nurses and midwives changed. All the money for the education of nurses and midwives has now been transferred to the NHSE. Up to this point, the Department for Education and Employment controlled the money for undergraduate programmes. Money for NMET is set aside (ring-fenced) by the NHSE from the annual NHS allocation, and this money cannot be used for any other purpose. The NHSE, in turn, divides the money between the education consortia according to agreed workforce numbers. Consortia are then able to contract competitively between universities to achieve the best value for money. The purchasing situation is different in Northern Ireland where education is purchased centrally by the Department of Health and where the sole preregistration education provider is Queen's University, Belfast.

Unlike the rest of the university sector, which relies upon money from the HEFC, with money allocated for a specified number of places (providing that quality criteria are met), health care education relies upon accurate planning of the future health care labour market. Places are determined by consortia, and contracts lasting for a 5-year period specify the number of students.

In postregistration education, money can come from two separate sources: the consortia, as the education meets predicted workforce need, and, of course, the student, who can opt to self-fund his professional development.

ACTIVITY 3.2

Contact the admissions office at your nearest university and that at a different university and ask for a prospectus dealing with a particular course in which you are interested (for example, intensive care or a Diploma in Professional Studies in Nursing). Compare the cost, mode and pattern of study. Decide which course might be right for you.

You may have based your choice on cost. Did you find much difference between the two centres? Or you may have preferred one option to another because the teaching programme coincided with your work pattern. The cost of a postregistration course is not always the greatest influence on choice – likes and dislikes also come into play. The marketing of education courses has rapidly assumed prominence to persuade students to buy.

Now focus on the cost of the course and compare it with the price of a domestic product, such as a dishwasher, or a luxury. How much of a diamond ring or motorbike will it buy? How will you estimate value for money with such an intangible product as learning, the success of which depends upon you as a student? What difference would this course make to your finances in terms of outgoings? Will you profit, in terms of enhanced salary or career prospects, at the end? Is it worth it? What difference will it make to the care that you give and the work that you do? Again, you can see that the individual purchasers deal with the same principles as an education consortium.

THE STUDENTS IN NURSING AND MIDWIFERY EDUCATION

ACTIVITY 3.3

From the students working in your clinical area at present, conduct a survey of their profile, including gender ratio, age, entry gate used, past experience, lifestyle and commitments.

You will no doubt have found a wide range of characteristics: graduates undertaking a shortened course, traditional 18-year-old 'A' level candidates, people entering with National Vocational Qualification (NVQ) level 3, nursing assistants who may have taken an aptitude test administered by one of the National Boards. You will guess from this rich mix that the challenge of getting the level of teaching and learning at the right level for everyone is daunting. Some of you may remember, not so long ago, the time when a married female student would have had to discontinue training. You may wonder how mothers with four children manage, but you will find plenty of them studying and sticking out the 3-year programme.

In 1985, there were more than 71 000 nursing students, and by 1996 this figure had dropped to 47 000 (Royal College of Nursing, 1997). This, together with the reduction in the number of nurses on the UKCC register and the ageing profile of the nursing workforce (with a disproportionate number due to retire between 1998 and 2003), presents a worrying trend in terms of nursing shortages. It poses a real issue for the workforce planners in terms of management of the shortages and of the recruitment of nursing students.

The age profile of nursing students in Royal College of Nursing (RCN) membership shows an average age of 26 years. Nursing students enter nurse education from a wide variety of backgrounds and non-traditional entry routes. Students are increasingly entering from another career with a wide range of experiences. The majority of students tend to be female, and there seem to be regional differences (Institute for Employment Studies, 1997). The Institute for Employment Studies' survey characterises the profile of nursing students; in Wales, for example, there appear to be a number of mature entrants to nursing from the mining community. There also appears generally to be an increasing number of students with dependants, and many are single parents. This poses a considerable challenge to study, shift patterns and clinical placements.

Some of you will have entered nursing from what used to be considered an exceptional pathway, but most of you probably entered nursing through the once-traditional route and may well spend some time wondering how child care or a mortgage can be paid for with a student nurse bursary. Consider also the strain that this may impose on an already challenged lifestyle and family and caring relationships.

TYPES OF PREREGISTRATION PREPARATION

Preregistration nursing education is currently offered along two pathways (Figure 3.4). The academic level of each course is different, although each prepares

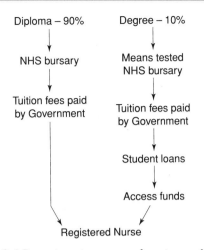

Figure 3.4 Preregistration nurse education pathways.

a registered nurse: one at diploma level, the other at degree level. Differences also occur in the funding and student financial support for each programme.

The diploma in higher education (DipHE) has always been part of the NHS workforce planning exercise, purchased through local education consortia according to projected workforce need.

Students receive an NHS bursary that is non means-tested and is (at current figures) approximately £5000 per year, depending on the age of the student, the number of dependants, whether the student is a lone parent or whether he is living in London, where a slightly higher award is made. Students in receipt of a bursary are not entitled to additional social security payments, including such things as housing benefit, income support and sickness benefit. If the student becomes ill for a long period of time, the bursary is suspended, but there is no entitlement to sickness benefit unless he formally withdraws from the course. Thus glandular fever or a similar condition can seriously affect a student's career plans and security. Tuition fees for nursing and midwifery are met by the purchaser. Ninety per cent of preregistration students are enrolled for a diploma in higher education.

Graduate course entrants in nursing at present account for 10% of the student body. Nursing degrees were developed during the 1960s to prepare academics, researchers and leaders of nursing. From 1998, degree students have started to be entered into the workforce planning exercise. Students receive a means-tested NHS bursary, and tuition fees are paid for by the NHS. The bursary is at the same rate as local government grants, and the same rules apply, so parental or partner income is a factor in eligibility. Undergraduate student nurses are not eligible to claim social security benefits but are able to access student loans and access funds. If a bursary is awarded, it is likely to be around £2000 per year.

There is no doubt that the move to provide both diploma and degree students with a bursary from the NHS is a move towards parity between the two groups, but differences in equality still remain. If a student loan is taken out by an undergraduate, this will have to be repaid from the April after the course has finished. The rate of interest equates with the rate of inflation, but repayments can be deferred when an individual's personal income is low. A loan may be the only means of survival for a nursing student, and the repayment may continue to represent a hardship issue for many years after registration.

At present, diploma courses form the majority of programmes purchased for preregistration nurse education. There are more degree applicants than available places and the provision of NHS bursaries could further influence this. In England, there was a shortfall of 1000 students for available diploma places, while there were 2000 more applicants for degree courses than places available (English National Board for Nursing, Midwifery and Health Visiting. 1997). This, coupled with the move towards a graduate nursing workforce, is likely to change the ratio in the commissioning of places between the two courses.

You may also have realised that hardship significantly affects the learning experience of many student nurses. Students' anecdotes indicate that student nurses spend 60% of their average income on accommodation. The RCN (1996), in a small survey, found that accommodation costs for students varied from university to university. If costs for books, food, social life, clothes, gifts, travel, heating and so on are added, it is obvious that the potential of the bursary is limited. Many students work as care assistants for a nursing bank or an agency, or undertake part-time work that is not linked to care. Recently, in a session with some nursing students, a speaker reported that a significant percentage of the group had worked during the previous night or had undertaken a twilight shift between two study days to support themselves – not an ideal learning experience.

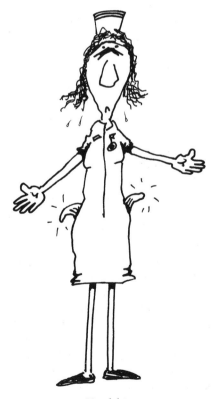

Hardship

The Dearing Report (DfEE, 1997) may move some way towards alleviating hardship by proposing to:

■ double higher education access funds for students in financial difficulty
■ allow students access to social security benefits
■ undertake an annual review of the total level of student living costs, taking into account the movement of both prices and earnings
■ withdraw student grants and replace them with student loans.

The difference between nursing students and those in mainstream education is in some ways obvious. Nursing students may require accommodation for 52 weeks of the year, particularly if they have dependants. The nature of practice placements also means that students need to work longer than the average 40 weeks per student year. Some nursing students are required to vacate the university halls of residence during traditional academic breaks, particularly the summer, when they are often on clinical placements. Nursing students receive payment for travel to and from clinical placements but not for commuting to the university premises. Travelling costs to universities can be considerable, particularly where amalgamations of colleges have taken place.

Although the nursing student's status in the practice setting is supernumary, many now believe that they contribute significantly to nursing care, and that if they did not do so, a replacement employee would have to be paid for, particularly at nights and at weekends.

The longer academic year, shift work and the demands of study limit the amount of extra income a student can earn, but there have been some extreme examples of students working all hours in order to stay the course. Although life for the nursing student has changed dramatically with the advent of diploma preparation, there are still many obstacles to overcome.

POSTREGISTRATION STUDIES

Post-registration studies clearly fall under the umbrella of lifelong learning, and educational activity at this point falls into two camps.

First, there is the continuing professional development that is required for periodic re-registration with the UKCC. Some Trusts make provision for nurses to attend study days in conjunction with the local university. Here, educational events are arranged that are linked to the practice of the nurse and to the achievement of their personal objectives and those of their Trust. Study days or educational events like this are not credit rated in the credit accumulation and transfer (CATS) scheme. However, the university will often seek a quality hallmark to ensure that standards are maintained. This may result in a rating that reflects student effort and hours of study, and reassures the university that quality assurance is maintained, as is seen in the accreditation granted by the RCN.

The second pathway that postregistration study lends itself to is to follow credit-rated courses that slot into the CATS scheme. Consortia may purchase courses with a specialist focus, for example, in caring for clients in the community or caring for older people. Courses are usually bought in bite-sized modules, each of which is CATS rated. The module may comprise weekly sessions or be offered in block form and will be pitched at academic level 2 or 3. As the student collects CATS points, he is working towards achieving a degree. Many students pursue several modules simultaneously, with a ceiling of three for part-time study. Within a degree pathway, there may be core modules common to a range of courses; an example of this is a research module. However, when a course is contracted by a consortium, it is normally focused at a particular set of insights and skills.

Postregistration nursing and midwifery courses offer a range of rich and rewarding opportunities that are often linked to CATS points. They also bring considerable personal and professional challenge.

INTEGRATING THEORY WITH PRACTICE

Nursing is a practice discipline with a strong tradition of learning by doing (National Health Service Executive 1997b). Until the 1960s, the responsibility for teaching nursing practice was vested in the ward sister. A new syllabus of training, which became operational in 1962, prescribed a strong theoretical base to nurse training, and this move probably coincided with the evolution of the theory–practice gap (National Health Service Executive, 1997b). Nurse tutors (as they were then called) taught theory in the classroom, and the sister taught practice in the ward. This brought about a potential disparity between what was taught and what was practised, causing conflict for nursing students, who tended to write one account of nursing for theoretical assessment and practise another in the clinical setting. Three pieces of research highlighted this problem (Alexander, 1983; Bendall, 1975; Gott, 1984). If you have not read these nursing classics, it is worth stopping at this point to borrow one and to compare what happened then with what happens today.

In the 1960s, clinical teacher posts, intended to reduce the theory–practice gap that was being increasingly documented, were created. Fretwell (1982), however, describes how the clinical teacher fell between the roles of ward sister and nurse tutor, lacking authority in both the ward environment and the school of nursing.

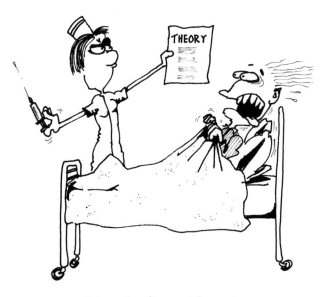

Integrating theory with practice

In 1980, as a further attempt to eradicate the problem of linking and integrating theory and practice, a new role, called the 'joint appointment', was established (National Health Service Executive, 1997b). This role involved a nurse working between the school of nursing and the clinical area. In reality, the role-holders became exhausted trying to work in two full-time posts.

In Oxford, in the mid-1980s, the role of lecturer-practitioner evolved. Vaughan (1989) reports that the post brought together practice, management, teaching and research as a clinical expert and a practice teacher. In 1997, the Chief Nurse for England requested a report on the lecturer-practitioner role. This revealed that there is still a lack of understanding of the role and a lack of promotion of its value. The report links into the debate around advanced practice and the preparation of nurse teachers (National Health Service Executive, 1997b). Kirk et al (1997) conducted a study focused upon the professional and academic needs of nurse teachers. The study reflected the problems of maintaining clinical expertise, the most frequently cited difficulty being lack of time; many respondents reported no reduction in workload to help with this. Nurse teachers are expected to spend 20% of their time in clinical practice, and this move, which could help to integrate theory with practice, is clearly not practicable, and is continuing to cause conflict.

The integration of theory with practice is, perhaps, the greatest challenge that the practitioner as a teacher faces. For a student to perceive his learning as seamless, a skilled and talented workforce has been at work using all the teaching skills they possess. If a student sees a separation between theory and practice, a greater use must be made of mentoring, supervision, reflective practice and experiential learning as the means of reducing it.

The theory–practice gap is still an issue. Strategies outlined in Chapter 1 are designed to minimise the problem rather than pretending it does not exist. At a recent conference, an eminent professor of nusing denied the existence of the theory–practice gap, stating that effective teaching mitigates against its presence. The integration of theory and practice poses a considerable challenge to everyone who interacts with students.

The report *Project 2000: Fitness for Purpose* by the University of Warwick (1996), highlights areas in which work is needed to improve the preparation of nurses, including at the interface between the university and the NHS. It also highlights issues around skills acquisition and the expectations of newly qualified nurses by employers. This qualitative study is one of the resources to be used by the UKCC in its review of preregistration education.

TEACHERS OF NURSING

Chapter 1 indicates that a teacher's role is varied and diverse. Figure 3.5 demonstrates the variety of roles that may be present in a lecturer's work. The richness of teaching is such that if you ask two lecturers to describe their work, you will gain two completely different accounts of its emphasis, of time allocation and of ways of working. However, both lecturers are likely to tell you that they undertake most of the activities in Figure 3.5 in varying proportions.

The prime function of a lecturer is to teach, either one to one in the university or clinical setting, or in lectures to a student body of 100 or so. As mentioned in Chapter 1, the type of teaching falls between two extremes that are best

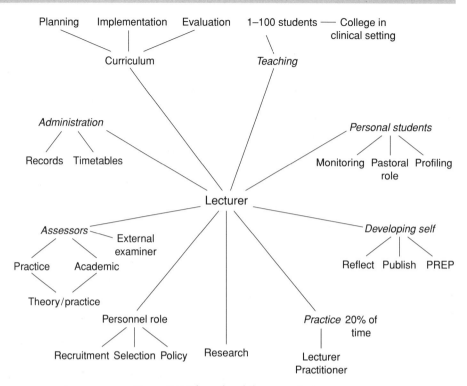

Figure 3.5 The role of the nurse lecturer.

summarised as the lecture at one end of the continuum and experiential learning at the other. Therefore, a lecturer's skills and self-awareness need to be expert. Teaching is just one aspect of the curriculum, but teachers also influence course design and evaluate and influence a programme as it progresses. The curriculum needs to evolve and grow as the needs of the client group change and social trends and technology influence a nurse's work and decision-making.

Personnel work is another important aspect of a lecturer's life as students and peers are recruited. Lecturers often contribute to the peer review of the department in which they work.

Increasingly, many lecturers are active in the field of research. Chapter 2 detailed the research assessment exercise, and many lecturers are engaged in individual and departmental projects that enrich and enliven their teaching, also producing publications and developing a profile in the research culture of the university. Research can originate from nursing practice and may even extend into research into successful teaching methods.

Most lecturers act as personal tutors to students, undertaking a pastoral role that ensures the student's well-being and also helping the student to make sense of his developing academic profile, enabling him to maximise his strengths as well as looking at ways of overcoming blocks and difficulties. This can be a demanding aspect of work, particularly when a student is not making good progress. Students span a wide range of ages, educational attainments, social and cultural groups and backgrounds. Their experiences are often diverse, and it is difficult to generalise from one student to the next. However, the personal tutorial role of the lecturer is both demanding and satisfying. Potential learning is two way – from student to lecturer and lecturer to student – a rich recipe when it works well.

Finally, for the lecturer to develop, it is important that he attends to his own profile, updating, meeting the requirements of postregistration education and practice (PREP), exchanging ideas and looking for ways of maximising strengths.

Lecturers usually work in a team, as shown in the academic profile in Chapter 2. Colleagues might include subject specialists from the worlds of sociology, physiology or psychology, as well as pure researchers, together with the mix of nurses from the family of nursing specialisms. Many nurse lecturers in higher education teach across a range of other courses as well as nursing, for example, psychology and health studies.

A survey conducted by the Association of University Teachers (1994) over a 2-week period demonstrated that the average length of the working week for academic staff was 53.5 hours, academic staff of professorial grade working on average a 59-hour week. The survey found that seniority brought an increase in administration and a decrease in the amount of time spent teaching undergraduates. Interestingly, the survey also reported that women worked longer hours than men, in particular in professorial grades, where women worked 65 hours a week on average, considerably more than their male colleagues. The survey also reported that women undertake a greater amount of administration.

The RCN (1993), in a discussion document, highlighted the changing world of the nurse teacher who leaves the NHS, changing employers to join the university sector, and the changing conditions of work that this brings. The discussion paper emphasises the importance of academic specialisation in specific subject areas, with future teachers of nursing working first and foremost as practitioners. The document, although in parts dated by recent changes in education, is still a relevant and thought-provoking read.

Prerequisites for teacher training

The UKCC is currently reviewing the process of becoming a nurse teacher and is working towards standards and outcomes that comprise broad sets of principles. These will allow institutions to offer adaptable and flexible pathways for teachers. However, nurse teachers are required to have a recordable teaching qualification on the UKCC register. The requirements of the teacher are listed in Box 3.2 Nurse academics are an all-graduate profession.

Teacher preparation is undertaken through postgraduate studies, and there are many flexible modes of study. Most are at postgraduate diploma level and

BOX 3.2	**Requirements for a teaching qualification on the UKCC register (United Kingdom Central Council for Nursing, Midwifery and Health Visiting, 1998)**

- A previous entry on the register at level 1.
- 3 years completed professional experience, normally with 2 of these spent in the UK in a post of responsibility involving the management of patient care. The nurse must also have experience in institutions where preregistration nurses are educated.
- Advanced professional knowledge to the level of a first degree in a relevant subject.
- A course of teacher preparation that must be approved by the relevant National Board.

carry CATS points towards a Master's degree, although some postgraduate certificates are offered. Many of the courses focus upon an interpretation of the role, i.e. as a lecturer–practitioner. A list of approved courses is available from the National Boards of each country.

It should be remembered that it is not uncommon for many lecturers to be recruited into the university sector because of their research profile and their ability to contribute to the research life of the faculty.

QUALITY IN NURSE EDUCATION

Many of the quality processes outlined in Chapter 2 apply to nursing and midwifery education. However, in the past, courses funded by the NHS have remained outside the quality processes of Quality Assurance Agency for Higher Education and HEFC. This will not apply to postregistration courses, for which the money for funding originates from the HEFC. Peer review of quality will still operate, and in courses that require approval by a National Board, conjoint validation schemes operate. This means that the normal validation panel is enhanced to include representatives from the National Boards. The National Boards have clear criteria that must be met if a course is to be given approval. Approval can be unconditional, for a period of 3–5 years, or it may be conditional upon certain requirements being met. In addition, a panel may make recommendations for a programme. The validation process is always supported by a detailed curriculum document, and conditional approval will usually require additional paperwork to demonstrate that the conditions have been met.

The panel will usually consist of internal and external assessors, the course team who have designed and will teach the programme, existing and prospective students, and members of staff from the clinical setting. In addition, academics from outside the department are usually present to ensure that university standards are met. A validation exercise is a rigorous, and often daunting, formal university process of peer review of quality.

CONCLUSION

The arrangements for nurse education are quite complex, and there are significant differences in the way in which our education system is structured and processed, as described in this chapter. The intention of this chapter has been to clarify and act as a resource that underpins the rest of the book. As such, there have been no reflective points, and only activities that are considered essential to grasping how things operate have been included.

This chapter ends, then, with a challenge – you may wish to reflect upon how the system has changed since you were a student, and then to consider whether you need to undertake any further activity to update your insight into the structure and system. You may wish to spend a day at the local university observing the recruitment and selection of future nurses and midwives. You may wish to work with a nurse teacher for a day, join a curriculum development group or a validation panel, or participate in some of the other activities that are part of everyday university life.

Finally, at the time of writing, there is a government Green Paper (a consultation exercise) on lifelong learning (1998) that builds upon the recommendations from the Dearing Report. The UKCC will shortly announce the standards for teacher preparation, which are likely to focus upon different levels of teacher preparation and include the preparation of mentors and teachers in the clinical setting, and the UKCC has also just announced a commision on the future of nurse education. Thus you will need to begin to make notes that will update this short chapter as these changes occur. In addition, you will need to read the news in the weekly nursing press to keep abreast of the changes. These are changing and exciting times, and you can exercise your right to participate in them.

GLOSSARY

Education consortia: regionally based groups that predict workforce needs and purchase education to meet the demands of health care.

Regional education development groups: there are eight of these in England, and they have an umbrella function over a number of consortia in the region.

REFERENCES

Alexander M (1983) Learning to Nurse. London: RCN.

Association of University Teachers (1994) Long Hours, Little Thanks. London: AUT.

Bendall E (1975) So You Passed Nurse. London: RCN.

Department for Education and Employment (1997) *Higher Education in the Learning Society*, (Dearing Report). London: Stationery Office.

English National Board for Nursing, Midwifery and Health Visiting (1997) *Annual Report*. London: ENB.

Fretwell J (1982) *Ward Teaching and Learning*. London: RCN.

Gott M (1984) *Learning Nursing*. London: RCN.

Humphries F (1988) Commisioning nurse education. *Nursing Standard*, 12(23), 45–47.

Institute for Employment Studies (1997) *Taking Part: Registered Nurses and the Labour Market in 1997*. Brighton: IES.

Kirk S et al (1997) Professional and academic needs of nurse teachers. *Journal of Advanced Nursing*, 26, 1036–1044.

National Health Service Executive (1997a) *Devolution of responsibilities to Education Consortia*. EL(97)30. Leeds: NHSE.

National Health Service Executive (1997b) *Lecturer Preactitioner Roles in England*. Leeds: NHSE.

Royal College of Nursing (1993) *Teaching in a Different World*. London: RCN.

Royal College of Nursing (1995) *A Principled Approach to Nurse Education*. London: RCN.

Royal College of Nursing (1996) *Nursing Student Accomodation Survey*. Unpublished document. London: RCN.

Royal College of Nursing (1997) *Response to Higher Education in the Learning Society*. London: RCN.

Scott P (1993) *The Transmission from Elite to Mass Higher Education*. Occasional Paper Series. London: Higher Education Division, DfEE.

Stock J (1996) Prepare to educate. *Nursing Management*, 3(7), 10–11.

United Kingdom Central Council for Nursing, Midwifery and Health Visiting (1988) *Criteria and Associated Guidelines for the Recording of Qualifications for Nurse Tutor, Midwife Teacher, Lecturer in Health Visiting, District Nurse Tutor and Occupational Health Teacher* PS&D/85/08. London: UKCC.

United Kingdom Central Council for Nursing, Midwifery and Health Visiting (1986) *Project 2000: A New Preparation for Practice*. London: UKCC.

University of Warwick (1996) *Project 2000 – Fitness for Purpose*. Warwick: University of Warwick.

Vaughan B (1989) Two roles – one job. *Nursing Times*, 85(11), 52.

FURTHER READING

Alexander M (1983) *Learning to Nurse*. London: RCN.
A classic research study that illustrates the theory – practice gap and offers the chance to compare the research findings with the present-day scenario.

Association of University Teachers (1994) *Long Hours, Little Thanks*. London: AUT. *Gives an insight into the life of higher education.*

Bendall E (1975) *So You Passed Nurse*. London: RCN. *Another brilliant example of the theory – practice gap.*

4 Assessing learning needs

Anne Eaton

INTRODUCTION

The word 'assess' is defined as 'estimate, magnitude or value or quality of' (*Little Oxford Dictionary*, 1989). In nursing terms, assessment can be defined as the means used to measure what students have learned. In this text, the 'learner' will be any member of the care team, within any care environment, who is on a course of study.

The term 'assessment' has different interpretations, depending upon the area of practice in which you work. All practitioners will be aware of the need to assess clients' needs, and most professionals will perform or contribute to this process in order to identify individual requirements, when planning care appropriately. This care, once implemented, can then be evaluated.

This process can now be matched to the learner in any care environment. The practitioner will come across many learners in their working lives, including nursing students, qualified nursing staff on postregistration courses, enrolled nurses undertaking conversion courses and health care assistants undertaking Scottish or National Vocational Qualifications (S/NVQs), and they all have learning needs, which will be individual according to their stage of development and their learning/ education programme.

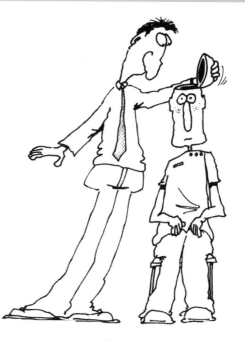

Assessing learning needs

LEARNING OBJECTIVES

After reading this chapter, you should be able to:

- assess learning needs
- devise a learning contract (action plan) with the learner
- implement, or help the learner to implement, the learning contract
- assess the learning that has taken place.

Encompassed within these four areas is also the notion that you need to be aware of the learning environment, the learning outcomes that the individual has to achieve and the methods of assessment that will best serve everyone's needs.

This chapter will include sections on the types of assessment that can be used in your learning environments, the notion of why, what, how and who to assess, and an exploration of the issues related to the learning environment. Learning contracts will be investigated, as will the use of reflection and reflective diaries. The best way to give feedback to learners will be explained, and the overall aim of the chapter will be to introduce and expand on issues of which you may or may not be aware in the field of assessment.

Assessment is a key component of every registered nurse's role. As previously suggested, qualified staff are confronted with a multitude of learners, and the process of assessment applies to all of them. However, despite the plethora of learners and their individual programmes, the processes of assessment are the same. The assessor needs to know and apply these principles across assessment situations and to individual learners.

TYPES OF ASSESSMENT

In educational terms, there are a number of types of assessment; some of these can be applied within the clinical environment, for example, your ward or department, but others apply purely to academic processes. As most of your students will be undertaking an educational programme, you need to be aware of the whole process that your students are going through, in order for you to piece together the jigsaw of theory and practice that will ultimately lead to the completion of a programme and a qualification, for example, as a registered nurse with a diploma in higher education (DipHE) or a degree in nursing.

Formative assessment

Assessment during a course or programme provides the means for the continuous checking of progress for both learners and teachers. This process fulfils a necessary formative function and serves to reinforce learning, confirming the learning that has taken place and highlighting the weak areas where improvement needs to take place. It can be likened to a 'mock' examination in which learning is assessed without the ultimate pass or fail grade, but giving feedback on progress to date.

In the assessment of theory, formative assignments, which may not be compulsory but depend upon individual learners' needs, are used to assess and monitor progress. At certain stages throughout courses, and at the end of some courses, the form of assessment may change and **formative assessment** then becomes summative.

Summative assessment

In the assessment of practice, you may use a continuous assessment strategy using formative techniques until you reach the stage at which you can confidently say that competence has been achieved and your assessment becomes final, that is, summative.

The **summative assessment** process often marks the end of one stage of the programme and the progression, or access, to the next phase. Within diploma level preregistration nursing programmes, the end of the common foundation programme (CFP) marks a summative assessment phase as this must be successfully completed before learners can move onto their chosen branch programme. For some educational programmes, the summative phase is used to grade the learners' outcomes, for example, with pass, merit and distinction grades, or a first- or second-class degree.

Norm-referenced assessment

This method is a way by which learners and their work and achievements are compared against those of other comparable learners and a norm is established. **Norm-referenced assessment** does not require that any overt learning objectives and assessment criteria be stated, nor is it a method that is transparent to learners or the staff involved (MADEN, 1997).

This process has many problems and is mentioned in this text so that readers can be aware of the method and its implications for a fair and honest assessment process. It can, for example, mean that a group of students may all be excellent and, using other methods of assessment, would all pass a particular assessment period well. However, using a norm-referenced process, they are compared against each other and only the very best pass. Alternatively, a group of learners may be equally poor, but the more able of the group pass because they are the best in a poor group.

ACTIVITY 4.1

Can you think of times when you have used norm-referencing?

You may think that you have never used this method, but perhaps the most common example of norm-referencing is when one nursing student is compared with another, even though the two may not have had the same experiences. This may be particularly relevant when comparing 'traditional' nursing students, who trained before the present-day diploma level courses, to students today, working for a diploma in higher education or a degree, when, in fact, no comparison should be made because of their different educational programmes.

Another example of norm-referencing may be when a nursing student is compared with a qualified nurse, when there is no comparison because of their very different experiences and expertise.

Criterion-referenced assessment

This method is a much fairer and more realistic assessment process and involves devising criteria that learners must achieve at certain stages of their programmes; they are therefore assessed against an independent standard. These criteria are the same for every learner at every stage in relation to the learning programme, so an objective assessment (i.e. one without bias) is made and the **validity** of the assessment is thus increased (MADEN, 1997). In terms of your involvement with learners, these criteria may take the form of learning objectives or outcomes and may be detailed in the course curriculum or, in the case of S/NVQs, laid down in the units of competence. In both cases, however, the outcomes are common to every learner, and some standardisation of assessment is therefore achieved.

Perhaps more importantly, **criterion-referenced assessment** provides a means of ensuring that learners achieve at least a minimum standard, important in the caring professions, including nursing, as a safety measure. This aspect is missing in norm-referenced assessment.

WHY ASSESS?

In many of the educational programmes in which you will be involved, for example, supporting preregistration nursing students, you will become involved in assessment because it is required by professional accrediting bodies, e.g. the United

Kingdom Central Council for Nursing, Midwifery and Health Visiting (UKCC), in their role as gatekeeper to entry into professional practice' (MADEN, 1997, p. 16).

In other words, assessment can be used to demonstrate the value, quality and standards of courses by measuring the learning of students who complete them. Ultimately, the UKCC is accountable for the complete process but you, as an individual assessor, are accountable for your own decisions when assessing learners.

The UKCC plays a key role in ensuring that new entrants to the nursing profession have undergone an appropriate educational experience and satisfied a certain standard of competence in theory and practice. It is your role to ensure that these standards are applied and adhered to in your area by the learners with whom you work. It can thus be seen that, through a variety of assessment processes, you, along with others, are ensuring that you produce competent practitioners, fit for purpose and fit for practice.

In the context of teaching and learning, assessment also provides feedback on the effectiveness of teaching. An important lesson to remember is that failure to learn is not always, or even normally, the fault of the learner, but can often be seen to be the fault of the teacher. In practice environments, assessors may also undertake the role of teachers, so this statement may refer to you!

ACTIVITY 4.2

Write down examples of 'good' teaching that you have experienced, which have enabled you to learn.

Write down examples of where you have failed to learn. Could this be attributed to poor teaching?

In my own experience, the best example I can give for good teaching is when I distinguished between 'hypo' and 'hyper', when related to, for example, blood sugar, when humour was used and 'hypo' was explained as what goes under and therefore 'hyper' as what goes above. I experienced bad teaching, in as much as I failed to learn, when the central nervous system was taught during my preregistration programme. This was because the topic was complicated and not made any easier to understand by the tutor as she did not relate it to physical conditions or nursing care.

If most learners fail in a certain aspect of learning, it may be because of the teaching process, and action needs to be taken to remedy this.

Feedback on learning

Feedback from assessment, whether the outcome is positive or negative, can often motivate the learner to progress, move on, maintain high standards or improve low ones. This is part of the formative assessment process and was discussed above. When you are assessing a learner for the first time, an initial assessment allows you, as the teacher and assessor, to find out what the learner knows, and this knowledge can then be used to form the basis of a learning contract.

On the whole, assessment should be a two-way process and ultimately a learning process for both the learner and the assessor. Both parties should be prepared to alter their practices according to the feedback that the assessment provides.

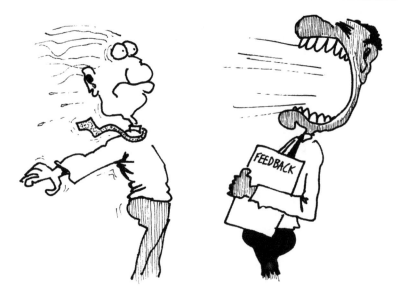

Feedback on learning

ASSESSMENT OF PRIOR LEARNING

Within current educational and employment practices, it is becoming increasingly necessary to recognise and credit learning that has already taken place in order not to repeat unnecessary learning experiences. In order to fit previously acquired knowledge and skills into a new programme, the learner can produce a portfolio of evidence, have aspects accredited and often be given a credit rating. The learner can thus be exempted from certain modules/ units in the new course. This makes educational (and economic) sense as it means that learners do not have to 'jump through the same hoop twice.' Instead, they can consolidate their existing knowledge and skills, and sometimes complete a programme of learning in a shorter period of time. Universities have all developed individual credit accumulation and transfer systems (CATS) in which components of learning are given credits within academic frameworks, for example, 30 credits at level 2 or 60 credits at level 3 (see Chapter 3). Unfortunately, there are problems with this system as some universities do not recognise or acknowledge the credit ratings awarded by other universities, making the term 'transfer' something of a misnomer. However, the system allows for individual and unique approaches to learning to occur, and for educational programmes to be tailor made to fit the individual and the educational establishment concerned. It is hoped that, in the future, institutions of higher education will be able to work towards a common tariff with regard to the transfer of credit.

ASSESSING LEARNING NEEDS

You will be aware of the diversity of learners in any care environment and of the fact that you, as a teacher and assessor, may be expected to be involved with all learners. This can be a confusing process, as most learners will be at different stages in their learning and will come armed with a plethora of paperwork. However, the processes of assessment are the same for all learners.

Time management of the assessment process is crucial to achieve positive outcomes. Some learners (for example, preregistration nursing students) may be with you for a very short period of time so it is vital that best use is made of this and your valuable contribution to their learning.

At the outset of their experience, you and your learner(s) need to identify specific issues:

- what learning they have achieved to date
- their personal learning needs
- the learning outcomes to be achieved during the placement
- planning for future learning.

The information gathered will enable you and your learner to develop a learning contract.

LEARNING CONTRACTS

The definition of contract is 'a written or spoken agreement', and in this case, the parties to this agreement are you, as the teacher and assessor, and the learner. Although the definition suggests 'spoken', it is generally advisable for the agreement to be documented so that both parties, and indeed anyone else (for example, the nursing student's tutor or the health care assistant's internal verifier,) who may need access to the contract, can examine the documentation.

Indeed, Richardson (1987, p. 202) describes a learning contract as 'a written agreement between teacher and student which makes explicit what a learner will do to achieve specified learning outcomes.' Box 4.1 shows an example of a learning contract drawn up between the two relevant parties – the assessor and the learner.

BOX 4.1	*An example of a learning contract*

Name: *Brenda Freeman*
Date: *10th June 1998*
Education programme: *NVQ level 3, care*
Care environment/ward: *Ward 9, Gynaecology*
Development/experience to date: *Previous general surgical experience*
Length of placement: *Permanent member of staff*
Assessor/mentor: *Anne Wilson*
Tutor/internal verifier: *Brian Szenawski*
Learning needs:
Individual: *To learn more about the care of patients needing surgery*
Placement: *To assess the competence of existing skills*
Programme/educational learning outcomes: *To complete the collection of evidence for unit Z19, undertake agreed clinical activities*
Methods of assessment: *Direct, live observation. Oral questioning, witness testimonies*
Expected date of achievement: *28th July 1998*

Interim review date: *2nd July 1998*
Signatures: Learner
B. Freeman
Assessor
A. Wilson
Date: *10th June 1998*

ACTIVITY 4.3

Select a learner, discuss with her the points made above and document your findings in the form of a learning contract.

A learning contract focuses on the process of learning rather than solely on the product of the learning process. Learning contracts are not new, although over the past few years, they seem to have achieved a more formal status. It has been suggested by Reed and Proctor (1993, p. 32) that 'Learning contracts have found a place in nurse education as they facilitate the development of independence in learners and practitioners.' One of the main advantages to a learning contract is its flexibility (Lowry, 1997).

Although it has been suggested that the contract is documented, it is not written in tablets of stone, and it can be altered to suit needs and circumstances. The important part is that these needs and circumstances are identified and incorporated rather than being seen as a hindrance to the process. Another, perhaps more important advantage, is that they may motivate learners to learn.

Dart and Clarke (1991) also suggest that learning contracts help learners to develop habits related to lifelong learning. The current educational processes for many of today's learners encourage, and indeed expect them to be autonomous individuals in charge of their own learning, and the use of contracts fosters that autonomy. The ownership of learning becomes a reality, and individual learning is the result. This can be a difficult concept for some practitioners to accept; the feeling of 'not being in control' can be overwhelming, but gone are the days when learners were spoon-fed knowledge and expected to absorb it at the same rate and with the same ability. However, according to McAllister (1996, p. 203), 'teachers should not deny their teaching and learning expertise and so should continue to advise, guide and encourage students to meet their learning objectives'.

In clinical practice, a learning contract can be used to bring theoretical learning into the practice setting and to enable the learner to apply her knowledge base within the practice setting, that is, to patient/client care. Nursing education is constantly criticised for the gap between theory and practice, and by using learning contracts, you are helping to close this gap by helping the learner to identify the links.

ACTIVITY 4.4

Identify an area of learning that became 'real' for you when applied in the practice setting. For me, this was when I was taught injection technique using an orange and then tried it on a real patient.

A warning may be necessary here; although we want to encourage learners to develop according to their own needs and identified outcomes, we must also ensure a degree of realism within the learning process and help them to set realistic and achievable goals.

OBJECTIVE-SETTING

Three areas will need to be taken into account in this context: the learners' needs, the assessors' needs and the course/programme needs.

Learners' needs

The learners' needs may include new skills and knowledge, and also revision and reassurance in relation to other areas that have already been experienced and assessed. The need here is to ensure that the learner can transfer existing knowledge and skills to new care settings and complete the cycle of learning.

In order to make effective use of a new learning situation, learners will need to know what can be learned in a particular placement. This is not quite as straightforward as asking them what they want to learn; indeed, this can be an exceedingly frustrating question. The learner needs to make an informed choice in order to plan her own learning needs, matching them with what the specialism has to offer. When you buy a new suit, you know generally what is on offer but not specifically what will meet your requirements. Likewise, in a new care/learning environment, a learner accepts that there will be staff, patients/clients and a certain type of experience to be gained, but does not know specifically what is available to extend her learning.

A word of caution is needed here as you have probably experienced learners who have identified too many learning objectives, and who want to 'run before they can walk'. This may be because the learner has identified a number of gaps in her learning and wants to fill them in one go, or because, according to McAllister (1996, p. 202), students may share a common and irrational belief that 'to be a registered nurse one must know everything about the principles prior to commencing practice'.

Assessors' needs

The assessor (i.e. you) needs to enjoy the teaching and assessing role in order to do it well. Time is often cited as a limiting factor when teaching and assessing learners in any clinical environment, and there is unfortunately no magic wand to be waved that will 'resolve' this problem. Therefore, assessors, their managers and learners have to be realistic about the needs of assessment, balanced against the other demands on their time. However, you also need to be aware of pressures put upon the learner, especially when her placement with you is for a short period only.

Realistically, assessing on a one-to-one basis is the method of choice, but this is often not appropriate, and you may need to supervise and assess a number of learners. Some of the problems associated with this can be overcome by utilising a shared learning contract, discussed below.

The assessor knows the learning opportunities that are available within the specific area and will need to make the learner aware of these opportunities in order that the optimal mix of learning objectives can be achieved. It is best to meet with your learners as soon as their placement begins, or before that if possible. Indeed learners may be encouraged to contact you prior to the commencement of the placement in order to start the familiarisation process. Ideally, you need to allocate approximately 30 minutes to commence the identification of the learners' and assessors' needs, but the use of this time should be well structured and profitable. As suggested, you need to help learners to identify what they need to gain from this particular experience, and your expertise and know-how will prove invaluable.

Course needs

The educational/learning programme that the learner is undertaking will almost certainly identify some specific and general areas of learning that must take place, and these must be taken into account when completing the learning contract. These areas of learning may be unique to a particular module or unit, and, in some circumstances, this will be the only opportunity for the learner to be exposed to this experience.

On the other hand, the general areas of learning may relate to common themes that thread through the whole of the curriculum or learning programme but which nevertheless need to be assessed in order to ensure that the learner can transfer and apply these to specific care situations.

ACTIVITY 4.5

Make a list of learning outcomes/opportunities that are specific to your clinical area and another list of general learning outcomes.

Your specific list may include, for example, the care of a patient requiring gastrostomy feeds or the communication skills involved in dealing with a suicidal patient in a mental health unit. Your general list may include the skills involved with the administration of medication or the completion of documentation needed when a new patient/client is admitted.

The latter two examples are areas of learning that apply in all clinical areas, which incorporate skills and an extensive knowledge base, and which the learner needs to apply consistently and competently across all care environments.

Whatever the detail of the contract, the content of it must be achievable and realistic, measurable at the end of the placement and, especially in the case of general objectives, transferable into the next learning context.

There is a possibility of devising a 'shared' learning contract between learners at the same stage of their learning processes. This may, in reality, be quite difficult. After all, we are all individuals and require holistic care, whether we are in a care setting or a teaching situation. However, when, for example, two or more health care assistants are undertaking the same unit for assessment within an S/NVQ award at level 2 or 3, parts of the learning contract will be common to each learner and therefore common to each learning contract. This can obviously be applied to other learners pursuing common programmes. The advantages are that the commonality will encourage and promote discussion, lead to shared learning and, in some circumstances, ease the burden of assessment on the assessor, as shared learning may mean that the learner partners support each other rather than expecting all their support from the assessor. Alternatively, you may be aware that this method may potentially increase your workload as the extra stimulation it offers may extend the learning process.

Similarly, it may be appropriate for an assessor in a specific and perhaps specialised area of practice to identify the learning objectives for every learner and to make these objectives the basis around which the remainder of the learning contract and objectives are devised.

RESOURCES

As shown in the example of a learning contract in Box 4.1, it is important to identify the key personnel involved. It is also important to identify other resources that will make the learning contract become 'live'. These resources may include other key individuals specific to the learning contract, for example, specialist practitioners, personnel outside the immediate environment, the patient's family and, of course, the patient himself.

'Hard' resources may include access to reference materials, case notes and research materials. Unfortunately, especially in relation to nursing students and postregistration learners, library facilities may well be housed within the formal learning environment, which may be a university some distance away from the placement, and forward planning and flexibility of access are vital if the identified learning is to take place.

COMPETENCE

We seem to expect more and more of our learners in relation to the amount and depth of knowledge required and the skills they have to perform in ever-expanding and more demanding care environments. These two components (knowledge and skills) must not be separated, whether you are assessing a health care assistant undertaking an S/NVQ at level 2 in care, or a preregistration student. The definition of **competence** appears to vary according to which text you are using and which learner you are assessing. Within care environments, the definition of competence must encompass the application of knowledge to skilled care delivery.

ACTIVITY 4.6

Without referring to any text, complete *your* definition of competence.

How did you express this? It is likely that your definition had something to do with skills or activities that are related to your job. You might like to compare this with the Manpower Services' (1981) definition as 'the ability to perform the activities within an occupation'.

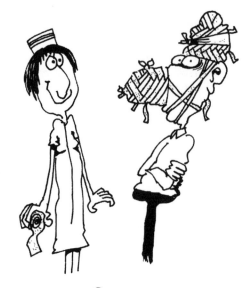

Competence

A definition of competence-based assessment is: a method of assessment that is developed from a set of general and specific outcomes, so that all concerned with the process can make fair and objective judgements about what the learner has achieved or not achieved, and that states student progress on the basis of demonstrated achievements of these outcomes. Assessments are not tied to a specific length of time spent in formal education (Wolf, 1995).

ACTIVITY 4.7

Apply this definition to:
- preregistration education programmes
- postregistration education programmes
- S/NVQ programmes.

In your opinion, does it fit all of these programmes well?

You may have identified such points as the clarity of outcomes within S/NVQ programmes and perhaps the different interpretations put onto some outcomes within preregistration programmes, which might not then fit the definitions of competence given earlier. You might also have noted that it depends upon the postregistration programme as to whether the definition fits the programme.

From the above definitions, you can see that achievement is measured against specific learning outcomes or objectives, all of which will be incorporated into one or more learning contracts and subsequently assessed.

METHODS OF ASSESSMENT

As can be seen by the definitions of the word 'competence', you may need to use a variety of assessment methods in order to encompass the whole concept and its diversity. You may argue that the knowledge base will be assessed through formative and summative assessment processes, usually written assignments and projects set and marked (assessed) by staff from the educational institution. While this may be correct for a number of learners, it is, as stated earlier, your role to help the learner to make concrete links between theory and practice, and you are a vital link in this chain.

The methods of assessment you can use with your learners in order to achieve the objectives laid down in the learning contract will include direct observation of performance, which can in itself indicate whether a learner is applying previously or newly acquired knowledge to practice. This link can further be confirmed through questioning, both informally after performing some particular aspect of care delivery, and more formally in an individual or group seminar or tutorial.

The use of direct observation provides evidence of development and progress, and an experienced assessor can assess much more than practice through the medium of observation. Indeed, this is a key method of assessing the application of theory to practice.

ACTIVITY 4.8

Think back to your days as a learner (which may be very recent). How were you assessed? List the good and bad points in this process.

You may have suggested that the best processes were when you felt well prepared for the session and the assessor was unobtrusive. I remember a time when, as a very new student, I realised that the ward sister did not necessarily need to see me work but could hear my actions and words from behind closed curtains!

The bad points you may have listed could include an inappropriate assessor, poor timing and not being personally prepared.

There are a number of ways of using observation as a method of assessment: as a 'one-off' and often planned process in which one specific component of learning is assessed in a series of prearranged sessions, such as when a unit from an S/NVQ is assessed; or in a continuous assessment process where the assessor is constantly, both directly and indirectly, watching (and listening to) the learner in normal day-to-day activities, formulating an overall holistic picture of the learner's development. These methods tend to indicate that the latter process gives a truer picture of the learner. We can all give an excellent 'one-off' performance, but in the competent practitioner there needs to be consistency in care delivery, which meets the learning objectives and, more importantly, the patients'/clients' needs at all times. A point to note is that 'if the learner can do it once, it's an event, twice may be a coincidence, three times may show that a consistent pattern is emerging,' (Stoker, 1994, p. iii).

You must not distance yourself entirely from the 'formal' written assignment or project that the learner may have to produce while working in your placement area. Indeed, the learner may identify you as the resource that makes particular areas of knowledge become 'live'. These assignments are almost always set by the staff within the institution where the educational programme is based, so, in the case of preregistration nursing students, assignments will be set by the lecturers in the university, and it will be a combination of contributions – yours included – that leads to a satisfactory outcome.

Other components of learning that can be taken into account by an assessor when forming an overall picture are the various documents completed by the learner, for example, care plans and fluid balance charts. Importantly, the one piece of evidence that might indicate a good standard of care delivery is a satisfied patient whose care needs have been met.

Whatever course or programme your learner is undertaking, you may at times need to assess a specific component of a learning contract or a specific learning objective. Equally, you may have to assess the learner through a myriad of learning experiences and processes leading to the assessment of the end result. For example, you may be required to assess whether a preregistration nursing student can manage the complexities of taking a patient's blood pressure, including having and applying the knowledge base related to the skill, or you may need to assess, over a period of time, how a learner cares for a patient admitted for surgery from admission through to discharge. This latter example will obviously take longer and will include the assessor taking into account not only concrete observable evidence, but also hidden skills. Stoker (1994) identifies four broad groups of skills which you will make decisions about (assess) the learner (Box 4.2).

BOX 4.2	*Stoker's (1994) four groups of skill to assess*

1. *Practical skills:* the ability to use equipment and carry out actions
2. *Intellectual skills:* related to knowledge and how the learner applies this, and concerned with activities such as planning, identifying priorities, problem-solving and decision-making
3. *Interpersonal skills:* the ability to communicate, form relationships and generally 'get on' with other people
4. *Intrapersonal skills:* concerned with the learner's self-confidence, self-control and awareness of her own abilities and the effect they have on others

ACTIVITY 4.9

Apply these four areas to the previous examples, that is, taking a patient's blood pressure and admitting a patient for surgery, and list the skills assessed.

You may have identified the following:

- Blood pressure:
  - practical skills: using the equipment properly, preparing the patient
  - intellectual skills: having the knowledge relating to the maintenance of blood pressure

 – interpersonal skills: talking to the patient
 – intrapersonal skills: the transferability of the skill to other situations.

■ Admitting a patient:
 – practical skills: preparing the bed, documentation, equipment
 – intellectual skills: understanding the need for accurate documentation, information-gathering, applying all the findings to the assessment of the patient's needs
 – interpersonal skills: talking to the patient, his family and other staff
 – intrapersonal skills: applying all the information to the whole process, such as preparation for theatre, consent to operation, physical care, information giving to the family and other carers.

Alternatively, devise an example of your own and identify the skills you will need in assessing the student. From these, it can be seen that your role as an assessor is not a simple one, and the role demands skills, such as the ability to remain objective, be realistic, communicate clearly, and perhaps most importantly, be truthful, offer and give feedback constructively, and document the result of the assessment process accurately. You have probably heard about, if not met, learners who seem to have completed a learning programme successfully but whose abilities appear lacking in practice. It is not easy to tell a learner that she has not been successful, but, from a professional point of view, assessors who are registered nurses are accountable to themselves, their employers, the profession and the UKCC for their practice, and they are accountable to their patients/clients in ensuring that whoever delivers care is competent and safe to do so.

You, as the assessor, may wish to use the learning contract and learning objectives as a checklist. In the overall assessment process, you and your learner must also be aware of the need to ensure that certain components of the evidence presented have been met (Box 4.3)

BOX 4.3	*Factors to ensure in the assessment process*

■ *The validity of the assessment.* That is, the assessment tool must measure the learning objectives it is intended to measure. For example, within an S/NVQ assessment process, assessment is based upon the competencies outlined in the appropriate units, elements and performance criteria (Day, 1996).

■ *The reliability of the assessment.* The assessment should produce the same results when used by different assessors or when used repeatedly with the same learner (Maden, 1997).

■ *The currency of the evidence.* The evidence, particularly written work that the learner produces, should be current, that is, up to date and relevant to the area/topic being assessed.

■ *The authenticity of the evidence.* Again, particularly in respect of written work, the evidence/work produced for assessment must be that of the learner and not someone else.

■ *The sufficiency of the evidence.* The assessor needs to ensure that she has seen, read or heard enough evidence from the learner for a clear decision to be made.

ASSESSMENT DOCUMENTATION

We have discussed learning outcomes, learning objectives and learning contracts in depth, but mention needs to be made of the forms and paperwork that you will need in order to document the results of your assessment processes. There are so many different kinds of documentation that it is inappropriate to give you an example of such a form here. You will have seen, or have access to, a variety of documentation, and it is your responsibility to make yourself familiar with the relevant forms. Remember, the job is not finished until the paperwork has been done!

However, regardless of the layout of the documentation, and of the course or programme for which it is intended, the key purpose of the form is for you to document the outcome of the assessment process so that the information is easily understood by other people and can subsequently be stored in the learners' records for reference at any time in the future. This is particularly important when external verifiers or examiners may be involved.

Key details that should be contained within the form include:

- the name of the learner
- the name of the assessor
- the name of the contact person, often a course tutor within the educational establishment
- the clinical placement/environment
- the dates of the placement
- the learning objectives as defined by the course/programme and by the individual, that is, the learning contract
- a means of documenting the outcomes of the process, such as 'tick boxes' or spaces for comment by both the assessor and the learner
- possibly a means of indicating which methods of assessment were used, for example, observation, questioning, written work or case studies
- spaces for the signatures and status of the assessor and learner
- the date on which assessment was completed.

ACTIVITY 4.10

1. Obtain existing assessment documentation.
2. Now devise an assessment sheet for a learning programme, unit or module that you assess which you feel improves upon the existing documentation. This might be for a preregistration student assessment, or a health care assistant undertaking an S/NVQ unit. Say how you feel your format is an improvement.
3. Suggest to the contact tutor that you might pilot test your revised form in practice.

Does your example contain all that is necessary for a third party, for example, an external verifier or examiner, to confirm and approve the assessment processes and outcomes?

As already suggested, there is no right or wrong way to lay out an assessment document. Criticisms around some processes, such as S/NVQ documentation, suggested that they were cumbersome and put excessive pressures on the assessors, while other forms appear limited and ultimately say nothing about the learner or what she has achieved. A happy medium clearly needs to be developed in all processes, and the S/NVQ documentation has gone through a complete review so that existing documentation has been changed in response to some of the criticisms.

You are key to the development of user-friendly and informative documentation, and your comments and feedback should be offered to those who devise the forms so that any necessary changes can be made.

LEARNING

When you are assessing a learner, you are looking for the evidence that learning has taken place and that this learning matches the learning objectives and the learning contract you have both developed.

It may be useful at this point to look at what learning is. The subject of learning theories will be covered in detail in Chapter 6, but you need to be aware of the ways in which individuals learn.

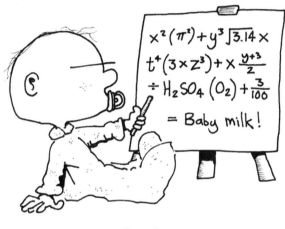

Learning

A definition of learning is 'knowledge got through study' (*Little Oxford Dictionary*, 1989), but in all definitions one component is common – that a change has taken place in the learner. Observing behaviour is a way in which you can detect such a change. Remember that just as you deliver holistic care to your clients, so should you treat your learners in an holistic manner, assessing them as a whole and not as separate parts.

ACTIVITY 4.11

List some of the ways you have learned in the past:

■ in school
■ in your preregistration nursing programme
■ in any postregistration programmes you have undertaken.

Which method do you prefer and why?

You have probably listed such examples as rote learning, as in learning and reciting the multiplication tables or poetry, learning through a teacher demonstrating a skill such as taking a patient's temperature, and self-directed learning, for example, using the library or studying by distance learning.

Your learners will probably give different examples, and they may cite varying preferences. For this reason, it is important to treat your learners as individuals.

WHAT TO ASSESS

The assessment process may vary in length and complexity according to the individual learner, the educational programme, the length of the placement and the learning outcomes/objectives to be achieved. It is ultimately the learners' achievements that have to be assessed, but overall the answer to 'What to assess?' can be encapsulated in:

- knowledge
- skills
- attitudes.

The first two areas are accepted by all assessors and teachers as the components of an educational or vocational programme. They are easy to define and relatively straightforward to assess, as they are 'concrete' for the assessor to see, and easy for the learner to demonstrate.

Attitudes can cause more concern as personal judgements can creep in and subjectivity can become problematic within the assessment process. Attitudes are, of course, highly individual. We are all different, so personal judgements about the attitude of a learner may differ from assessor to assessor. What must be identified are the attitudes that are necessary for effective practice in specific care settings, remembering that attitudes that are helpful in one area may not be appropriate in another. For example, it may be acceptable to be very informal with colleagues in a mental health unit in order to promote a feeling of normality, but that same approach may not be appropriate in an operating department. However, in all care areas, it is important to maintain and demonstrate respect for and the dignity of patients/clients at all times.

Having said this, it still remains important to assess attitudes as they encompass the notion of professionalism. Perhaps the best and fairest way to assess the attitudes of an individual learner is over time, in a number of situations, with feedback coming from a number of assessors and other personnel involved with the learner, so that a conclusion can be drawn on whether the learner's attitude fits the learning and workplace environment.

Remember that when learners join caring professions, some of them are very young, most of them are inexperienced and virtually all of them are, at some time, frightened about what they are doing. Appropriate attitudes are often associated with maturity, experience and confidence in ability, so the assessment of attitudes needs to span the whole of a learning experience, with feedback given as and when necessary, for example:

- throughout and at the end of a placement
- throughout and at the end of a module
- throughout and at the end of the CFP

ACTIVITY 4.12

Think of a learner you have worked with whom you considered to have an attitude problem. After working with you, did he or she go on to:
■ stay the same
■ change
■ complete his or her programme?
What was your opinion of the learner's progress?

so that the individual learns what is appropriate in different circumstances and at different times.

This leads to looking at how the individual learns from different experiences and uses these to develop the appropriate level of knowledge, fitting all learning opportunities together and reflecting upon the whole learning programme.

REFLECTIVE LEARNING

The use of reflection, often in the form of reflective diaries or journals, is becoming more widespread in nursing and, indeed, within education generally.

Reflection means looking back, thinking about what has happened previously and hopefully learning through and from those experiences. If you have read and worked through this chapter, you will (hopefully!) have used some of the activities interspersed throughout the text. In so doing, you will have reflected on some of your practices and those of others, and we hope that you will feel able to use your experiences to enhance and progress your learning. You have, therefore, used reflection as part of your learning process.

We all reflect, in our day-to-day and working lives. In the majority of cases, this reflection may be simply: 'I enjoyed that restaurant, and I'll go there again' or 'I could have performed that skill better.'

Within your professional role, and indeed to fulfil the requirements of the UKCC and their standards for postregistration education and practice (PREP) (United Kingdom Central Council for Nursing, Midwifery and Health Visiting, 1994), you will have to demonstrate how, over the 3-year period leading up to your periodic re-registration, you have kept yourself up to date. Additionally, you need to be able to produce documentary evidence of how, through reflection, your updated knowledge and skills have affected your care delivery. To meet the UKCC's requirements, you will need to keep a personal professional **portfolio**, which may well contain a reflective diary and from which you can draw an appropriate **profile** to demonstrate professional updating. Similarly, your learners, particularly nursing students, are encouraged or expected to keep and use reflective diaries throughout their educational preparation, whether on diploma or degree programmes.

This reflective diary can, and must, form part of your assessment tool as it will link the areas of practice and the experiences through which your learner has gone in a consolidated format. Andrews (1996, p. 508) states that, 'although clinical expertise in nursing is commonly accepted, in the main it receives less recognition than academic achievement'. There have been some attempts to

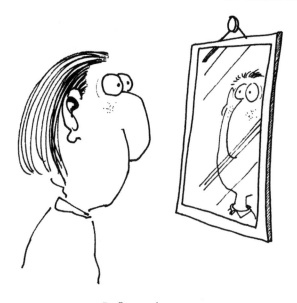

Reflective learning

redress this imbalance, and the ability to reflect effectively is fundamental to the development of nursing practice.

The format of reflective diaries ought to mirror the specific learning objectives and outcomes in order for the reflective diary to be an effective assessment tool. Furthermore, the English National Board for Nursing, Midwifery and Health Visiting (ENB, 1992) suggests that the adoption of learning diaries in the UK represents a move away from the concept of education as a product, towards emphasising nursing education as a lifelong process.

Although we have concentrated so far on the use of reflection on practice experiences through documentation in a diary, it is worthwhile noting that by discussing practice, either as an individual or in a group, learners can share their experiences, reflect upon their own and their colleagues' activities and therefore learn from each other's experiences. Comparisons can be made and a greater awareness developed of the contexts and diversity of practice, and the ability to apply principles of performance, identifying that, in some circumstances, there are no right or wrong ways to perform a skill, but a variety of methods that can be used. Through this process, we can continue to move the learners away from rote learning towards a more analytical process that includes problem-solving.

It can be suggested that, by assessing a learner's reflective diary through a formative process, there is scope for formulating strategies to offer developmental opportunities and enhance performance. When we looked previously at the assessment of learners' attitudes, we suggested that this needs to be done over time, taking different learning experiences into account. A reflective diary is a very useful tool that will contribute to the assessment of attitudes as it allows the assessor to see things from the learners' perspectives.

We have stressed in this chapter that objectivity of assessment is of paramount importance in achieving a true and realistic assessment of learners, but reflection, because of its personal nature, leads to a subjective documentation of occurrences and development.

ACTIVITY 4.13

Think back to when you were last asked to comment about *your* work, either as a student or as a practitioner. Did you give yourself a realistic assessment?

On the whole, learners have a tendency to be overly critical of their own abilities, so reflection may need to be somewhat tempered. When applied to nursing knowledge and the performance of skills, reflection becomes a learning tool and can be seen to be deliberate and purposeful, the aim being to change behaviour. By reflecting upon practice, a learner can think about why she performed activities in a certain way, decide whether the process was appropriate and potentially identify ways in which to improve on this performance.

The contents of a reflective diary may follow a particular pattern, which helps to give it a constructive format and enables its use by a variety of people. A word of caution is needed here as a reflective diary can be seen as a private and personal tool, and access by others may be restricted or not permitted.

The process could start with a description of an event, followed by the individual interpretation of feelings about the event. The next phase could involve the evaluation of the experience and be followed by an analysis of the situation, including thoughts about what else, if anything, could have been done. The final phase would be to develop a plan for future action should the same or a similar situation recur.

Confidentiality

As reflective diaries detail a learner's experiences, and these will obviously include patient/client care, they must, by implication, contain details about individuals. Thus, the issue of confidentiality arises. Learners must be made aware of the need to maintain confidentiality with respect to clients and colleagues, and to complete their diaries in such a way as to maintain the anonymity of all concerned.

In conclusion, it can be seen that reflection can contribute greatly to the learning process, especially learning through experience, and this experience, via the reflective diary, can then be assessed by you. The function of reflection and the use of reflective diaries as an assessment tool suggests that learners receive feedback about their practice from themselves and from you. Whatever is assessed and whatever the means of assessment, the learner needs to know how she is progressing, and this means that you need to give feedback in relation to her learning.

FEEDBACK

The feedback given during the assessment of reflective diaries is essential, but it should not be seen as the only occasion on which feedback is given. We all need to know whether we are performing well or whether there is room for improvement. This feedback applies not only to your learner, but also to you, as a lifelong learner, constantly consolidating and enhancing your knowledge and skills.

Feedback, therefore, is an important part of learning. Intrinsic feedback can be gained from performing a skill; that is, you sense in a number of ways that you have performed well, and the feedback is immediate. Extrinsic feedback comes from outside the learner, often from teachers and assessors. Within the sphere of care delivery, feedback on the acquisition of skills and knowledge is necessary at a number of stages:

- until mastery and expertise are achieved, in which case the feedback is formative in nature
- when mastery and expertise have been achieved, when the process is summative. It is necessary at this stage so that competence and standards can be maintained.

In both circumstances, feedback can motivate learners to continue and enhance learning.

So, how should feedback be delivered, by whom and when?

ACTIVITY 4.14

Think of a situation in which you were the learner. How did you know if you were performing well? How did you know if you were not performing well? Who gave you the information?

Your observations may include:

1. You knew you were performing well because:
   - you were complimented by other staff
   - you felt inside that you had performed well
   - your patient/client was grateful for your care delivery
   - you received a positive evaluation at the end of your course of study/learning
   - no-one commented when you did well, only when you performed badly!
2. You knew you were performing badly because:
   - other staff told you so
   - other staff avoided working with you
   - you knew inside that you had performed badly
   - you did not receive a good evaluation at the end of the experience.

From these examples, we can see that a number of people are involved in giving you feedback – other staff, patients/clients and you yourself. One point that needs to be stressed is that whoever gives feedback needs to do it in a constructive and positive manner. You are acting as an assessor to 'build' learners rather than knock them down. There is something positive to say about everyone, and learners will listen to and accept criticism if it is given in such a way as to be constructive.

Perhaps your response might be that you did not tell him or her but left the person to continue as before, in the hope that someone else would solve the problem, maybe even in another clinical placement. Think of the implications of this.

Think of a learner you have worked with who did not perform well. How did you tell him or her?

A positive and constructive way of giving feedback is as a 'praise sandwich'. By this, we mean that you start your feedback by giving the learner something positive to hear about her progress, then, if necessary, discuss the areas that need improvement in the middle, and then complete your feedback with another positive statement. An example of this approach is given in Box 4.4.

BOX 4.4	A 'praise sandwich'

Top slice: You did well in preparing the equipment and medication needed for Mr Carpenter's intramuscular injection.
Middle: 'However, I feel you could have improved your communication with him and given him a little more information about what you were giving him and why.'
Bottom slice: 'Your administration technique was good and you went on to reassure Mr Carpenter well following the procedure.'

Hopefully, by delivering feedback in this manner, learners will identify and maintain the good practice referred to in the feedback and acknowledge what they need to develop and improve in the future.

Of course, you have no problems if your learners perform well in all aspects, but these will be rare occasions. Having said this, all learners need to know how they are performing, even those who are doing well, and unfortunately these learners are often not told.

Do you think is it easier to give feedback about good work or bad work? When did you last do either?

As an assessor, you are a key player in informing the learner about her progress, that is, in giving feedback. You can do this orally, in a formal or informal discussion with your learner, or in writing, by completing the relevant assessment documentation. Although there may be limitations to what you can write because of the structure and format of the documentation, you may also be involved in marking written work that you or others have set for the learner. In this process, you can obviously give a mark, for example, 7 out of 10, or 65%, which does mean something to the learner but does not tell her which were the good and valid points, where she could have elaborated and extended the work or where there were errors. The solution to this is to write detailed comments, on the paper if possible or on a separate sheet, giving the learner positive feedback on the work. If you are involved with marking written work and giving feedback in this way, it is important that you do it fairly rapidly so that the work is fresh in the learner's mind and the comments can be acted upon and used to consolidate learning. Of course, in a practice setting, feedback needs to be immediate, especially if the actions of the learner might jeopardise patient/client safety.

As with the 'praise sandwich' approach, you need to document all your findings in a positive manner and try to ensure a 'personal touch'. That is, you refer to your learner as an individual with personal attributes rather than as one of many, remembering the comments made earlier in the chapter about 'norm-referencing.'

ACTIVITY 4.17

Perhaps the easiest way to illustrate this is to put yourself in the position of a woman telephoning the ward to ask about the condition of her husband, who is a patient. Would you prefer to hear: 'He is comfortable' or 'He is comfortable after a fairly good night's sleep, and he has just had some breakfast'?

A 'personal' touch goes a long way towards relieving anxiety and demonstrating that you know *whom* you are giving feedback about.

Throughout this section, we have suggested that feedback is part of the assessment process, but we will also see that feedback contributes to the evaluation process (see Chapter 7).

THE LEARNING ENVIRONMENT

Feedback is given about the learners' progress within a variety of clinical placements, but some areas appear to be more conducive to learning than others.

Most of your learners will find the clinical area a frightening place, and to begin with, learning will be limited. At the start of their educational programmes, nursing students spend a long time in a classroom environment, with only minimal exposure, as observers, to the clinical environment. Some learners may also experience difficulties in coming to terms with a specific ward or department; this includes newly recruited staff at all levels, from RGNs to health care assistants.

Your role will be to help the learners to settle into a new environment initially and then to enable them to use the area as a learning environment as their confidence grows. As already indicated in the section 'Why assess?' it is part of your role to enable the learner to link theory to practice, and the ward or clinical area is where this connection takes place.

According to Ogier (1989, p. 67), in order for learning to occur, the clinical area has to be managed by a leader who is in touch with the needs and abilities of her subordinates, and who is able to create an atmosphere which is conducive to learning. In reality, today's ward leader will have a diversity of roles to fulfil, but the importance of the role of teacher and the facilitator of learning must not be underestimated. With the support of the ward leader, other staff feel comfortable in taking on this role and developing the learning environment.

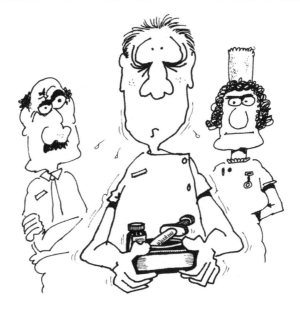

The learning environment

ACTIVITY 4.18

Think for a moment about what you consider to be conducive to the development of a good learning environment. Jot down the essentials.

Your list may include:

- a committed and enthusiastic ward manager
- a committed and enthusiastic ward team
- a manageable workload
- an appropriate level of staff who can teach and assess
- motivated learners of all kinds (but not too many)
- time to teach and assess.

The throughput of clients in all clinical areas, including acute and community NHS Trusts, is increasing, often with greater patient/client dependency. Consequently, staff are overstretched. However, we must make time for learning to take place in order to ensure that we prepare the practitioners of tomorrow – and the best place for learners to acquire clinical skills and to link theory to practice is the clinical environment. We cannot wave a magic wand to change our clinical environments, but what we must learn to do is manage time effectively so that appropriate space and effort can be given to supporting learners in helping them to learn. This does not necessarily mean one-to-one tuition. Learners can and must observe performance by **direct observation** and **indirect observation**; you act as a **role model**, and in so doing, you facilitate learning.

Learners not only identify and observe specific skills, but also observe your communication skills, your problem-solving and prioritising strategies, that is, not only what has to be done but in what order to do it, and your decision-making strategies. Thus, in carrying out nursing practice and acting as a role model, you are teaching all of the time, and it need not take 'extra' time. However, many nursing students, when on placement in a very busy clinical environment, may not realise what learning has taken place until this has been made explicit, discussed and analysed, and the links made.

Previous studies by Orton (1981) and Ogier (1982), although dated and set in the days when preparation for practice used an apprentice-type approach, examined whether nursing students viewed themselves as learners or workers. Although the nursing students today are involved in very different educational programmes, we may still need to ask the same questions.

Throughout a major part of preregistration programmes, nursing students are said to have supernumerary status, that is, they are not counted as part of the workforce, as pairs of hands; they are simply expected to observe care delivery. There does appear to be some discrepancy surrounding the role of the nursing student as some value this approach while others feel they want to get on with practising.

However, one thing is certain – that nursing students are in clinical placements to learn, and that this will differ according to their previous learning and experiences, and with the clinical environment.

Interestingly, the results of the two studies cited indicated that, after the first clinical placement, learners felt like workers for 80% of the time and learners for 64%, whereas at the end of the third year of training, they felt like workers for 100% of the time and learners for 34%.

We have thus identified components of the clinical environment that make it conducive to learning. In an ideal world, these would be as listed in Box 4.5.

BOX 4.5   *Characteristics of the clinical environment that make it conducive to learning*

- Good and effective links with the educational establishment, perhaps through a link tutor
- Dedicated and uninterrupted time for group and individual seminars and tutorials
- The use of the multidisciplinary team in the delivery of teaching and the assessment of educational processes
- Adequate resources in the clinical environment:
  - nursing publications
  - up-to-date text books, videos, etc
  - access to research relevant to the clinical environment
  - staff who undertake research and who can involve learners
- Dedicated staff, committed to enabling others to learn through a variety of processes and who have been adequately prepared to undertake the roles as teachers and assessors

THE STATUS OF ASSESSORS

All staff contribute to the assessment of both patients/clients and learners alike. The golden rule concerning who assesses what is that assessors must be competent in the skills they are assessing. Some may not need specific preparation for this role inasmuch as their opinion may be sought about the outcomes of a specific aspect of care delivery or the development of the learner, perhaps in relation to a specific learning objective or outcome.

In S/NVQ terms, this method of assessment, when applied to learners, is termed a 'witness statement' or 'testimony'. This entails an individual assessing an area of work – perhaps an element within a unit of competence – and making a written statement of the process and outcome for the learner to pass on to her 'official' assessor as a contribution to the assessment process.

ACTIVITY 4.19

List the staff whom you have involved in assessing learners or whom you could involve in the future.

Your list may include:

- registered nurses of all grades
- other professionals, for example, physiotherapists, occupational therapists, dietitians, speech therapists and doctors
- the ward clerk/receptionist
- the unit manager.

This is a healthy and useful mix of personnel and should lead to an objective and well-rounded picture of an individual learner. From the list above, you could identify, for your area, who would assess what.

Most educational establishments and the statutory/awarding bodies involved with nurse education will stipulate the specific preparation that assessors need to go through in order formally to assess a specific programme.

ACTIVITY 4.20

List the assessor preparation courses of which you are aware.

Your list will almost certainly include the ENB course 'Teaching and Assessing in Clinical Practice', commonly known as ENB 998, or its equivalent in midwifery practice – ENB 997. This may be delivered as a 'stand-alone' award or may be incorporated as a module into other programmes. For some of you, this programme may be neither appropriate nor available, as it is an *English* National Board course, and there may be equivalent programmes of study approved by your relevant Board or other educational establishments.

You may also have included in your list the Training and Development Lead Body (TDLB) assessor awards, commonly known as the 'D' units. These are two specific units of competence that S/NVQ assessors need to undertake to demonstrate competence in the assessment of these awards. Although these are generic awards, covering all S/NVQ assessment processes, it does not follow that once an individual has gained these awards, she can assess any S/NVQ. As previously stated, 'assessors must be competent in the skills that they are assessing' so care S/NVQs must be assessed by competent carers (not necessarily professionally qualified nurses). These awards, or rather the learners undertaking these awards, must not be assessed by any other S/NVQ assessor.

There are two assessor awards for people assessing S/NVQs, namely:

1. D32 – Assess Individuals' Performance. This looks at the role of direct observation in the assessment process.
2. D33 – Assess Individuals Using Different Evidence. This unit looks at other methods of assessment, such as oral and written questions, and, as mentioned earlier, witness testimony.

In both examples, that is, ENB 997/998 and D32/33, assessor candidates need to acquire the skills and knowledge to undertake the role and to demonstrate their competence in the role. Thus the assessor becomes the learner, and we have gone full circle. You may consider, in your future career, becoming more formally involved with nurse education, within an NHS Trust, for example, working within a training and development department, or within a university, possibly within a faculty of health.

Nurse education has gone through major reforms, the most recent being the introduction of diploma level preregistration programmes and the move into higher education, which, for Northern Ireland, was not completed until September 1997. These moves are discussed in detail in Chapter 3.

Potential employers of nurse educators, particularly in higher education, are looking for staff with clinical experience, an extensive knowledge base, potentially at Master's level or above, and an awareness of or involvement in research. Nurse educators are still relatively new and unusual within the world of higher education as they all have to be professionally qualified nurses holding a teaching qualification. This may alter in the future because of the recommendations contained within the 1997 Department for Education and Employment White Paper, *Higher Education in the Learning Society*, normally referred to as the Dearing Report (Department for Education and Employment, 1997).

The UKCC (1997) has undertaken a substantial piece of work to look at the standards for the preparation of nurse teachers, a topic examined in Chapter 2. The main themes include teachers as:

- mentors
- practice educators
- lecturers.

The standards will outline the preparation that these educators will be expected to undertake in order to move nurse education into the next millennium.

CONCLUSION

The assessment of all learners involved with the delivery of patient/client care, regardless of their educational programmes, is of paramount importance when you consider that, through the assessment of learning, you are contributing to the development of competent and safe practitioners and carers now and for the future. Assessment gives direction to both learning and the efforts of learners, and is a means by which the quality of an education programme can be demonstrated.

It can be a difficult role, it can be a time-consuming role and there can be internal conflict when informing a learner of an outcome that she does not want to hear, but, above all, it is a rewarding role, helping to develop staff with high standards, a sound knowledge base, a wealth of competence in skills delivery and the attitudes appropriate to dealing with complex situations.

This chapter has examined a range of issues, the most important of which focus on the accurate and objective assessment of individual learners, using a variety of methods, and the completion of clear and informative documentation.

Assessment strategies need to provide a balance between what is required, what is manageable and what is ideal, and this is now your role. Enjoy it.

GLOSSARY

Criterion-referenced assessment: assessment against a set of standards or criteria.

Competence: the ability to perform to an agreed standard.

Direct observation: in contact with; watching someone perform.

Feedback: informing the learner about achievements.

Formative assessment: ongoing assessment throughout the learning process.

Indirect observation: observation that is not direct; assessment using other methods, such as talking to other staff involved.

Norm-referenced assessment: assessment relating performance to that of a typical learner population.

Portfolio: a collection of evidence that demonstrates, for example, experiential learning, continuing professional development.

Profile: a collection of information that gives details of the individual concerned for a particular purpose.

Reliability: the consistency of assessment across assessors and assessment situations.

Role model: an individual whom a learner may choose to copy or model themselves on.

Summative assessment: a type of assessment usually used at the end of a period of learning.

Validity: how well a test measures what it is supposed to measure.

REFERENCES

Andrews M (1996) Using reflection to develop clinical expertise. *British Journal of Nursing*, 5(8), 508–513.

Dart B and Clarke J (1991) Helping students become better learners: a case study in teacher education. *Higher Education*, **22**, 317–335.

Day M (1996) *The Role of the NVQ Assessor*. Edinburgh: Campion Press.

Department for Education and Employment (1997) *Higher Education in the the Learning Society* (The Dearing Report). London: HMSO.

English National Board for Nursing, Midwifery and Health Visiting (1992). *The Development and Promotion of Open Learning Systems Project. Final Report*. London: ENB.

Little Oxford Dictionary, 6th Edition (1989) Oxford: Clarendon Press.

Lowry M (1997) Using learning contracts in clinical practice. *Professional Nurse*, **12** (4), 280–283.

McAllister M (1996) Learning contracts: an Australian experience. *Nurse Education Today*, **16**, 199–205.

MADEN (1997) *Guide to Assessment of Students' Progress and Achievements*. London: DfEE.

Manpower Services (1981) *A New Training Initiative. Agenda for Action*. London: HMSO.

Ogier ME (1982) *An Ideal Sister: A Study of Leadership Style and Verbal Interactions of Ward Sisters with Nurse Learners in General Hospitals*. RCN Research Series. London: RCN.

Ogier ME (1989) *Working and Learning*. London: Scutari Press.

Orton HD (1981) *Ward Learning and Climate. A Study of the Role of the Ward Sister in Relation to Student Nurse Learning on the Ward*. RCN Research Series. London: RCN.

Reed J and Proctor S (1993) *Nurse Education: A Reflective Approach*. London: Edward Arnold.

Richardson S (1987) Implementing contract learning in a senior nursing practicum. *Journal of Advanced Nursing*, **12**, 201–206.

Stoker D (1994) Teaching and learning in practice. *Nursing Times*, **90**(13), i–viii.

United Kingdom Central Council for Nursing, Midwifery and Health Visiting (1994) *Post Registration Education and Practice Project*. London: UKCC.

United Kingdom Central Council for Nursing, Midwifery and Health Visiting (1997) *Standards for the Preparation of Teachers*. London: UKCC.

Wolf A (1995) *Competence Based Assessment*. Milton Keynes; Open University Press.

FURTHER READING

Day M (1996) *The Role of the NVQ Assessor*. Edinburgh: Campion Press. *This text gives the ward-based assessor an insight into the assessment of NVQs and gives definitions of 'competence' that the reader can then compare with other definitions used outside the NVQ context.*

Kirk S, Carlisle C and Luker K (1997) The implications of Project 2000 and the formation of links with higher education for the professional and academic needs of nurse teachers in the United Kingdom. *Journal of Advanced Nursing*, 26, 1036–1044. *Although not directly related to the topic of assessment, this paper presents the findings of a national study relating to the impact of Project 2000 and the move into higher education. The research highlights the need for clinical credibility to be clearly defined in relation to to nurse teachers.*

Ogier ME (1982) *An Ideal Sister: A Study of Leadership Style and Verbal Interactions of Ward Sisters with Nurse Learners in General Hospitals*. RCN Research Series. London: Royal College of Nursing. *Although now a dated text, this gives the reader an insight into earlier research and allows the reader to compare how this relates to today's working environments. Indeed, it demonstrates that some issues do not go away.*

5 The process of learning

Sue Howard

INTRODUCTION

The aim of this and the following chapter is to provide you with the knowledge and skills needed to make your teaching effective.

Increasingly, as a practitioner, you are required to take on a much more formal teaching role. There are many reasons for this. It may be as a direct result of the increased autonomy of nurses, as identified in the United Kingdom Central Council for Nursing, Midwifery and Health Visiting (UKCC) *Scope of Professional Practice* (1992a), or of the specific needs of employers. In addition, the specialisation of many areas of nursing frequently means that the person most up to date with current developments in practice is you, the nurse providing the care. Intensive care nursing and renal nursing are clear examples of this, since the care required has become more complex, and the number of nurses able to fulfil the role are limited. It is, therefore, not surprising that, as a practitioner in nursing, you will often find yourself having to prepare and deliver educational material to a variety of audiences, from both within and outside the profession. This quite often causes a degree of anxiety when you feel daunted by the prospect of speaking to people on a formal basis in spite of the fact that you are the 'expert' in the subject.

There will undoubtedly be many more reasons why you may be reading this chapter. For example, it may be as part of a teaching course, as preparation for a teaching session or to find out how to maximise the learning experience for students in practice. Whatever the reason, it is necessary to understand the current thinking on how learning takes place if teaching is to be effective. This involves the ways in which we learn.

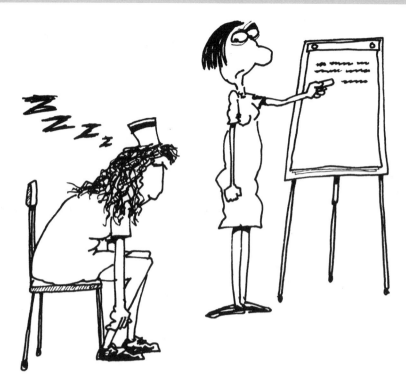

The process of learning

LEARNING OBJECTIVES

After reading this chapter, you should be able to:

■ discuss the interdependent nature of teaching and learning

■ recognise the importance of individual differences in the learning process

■ identify the learning theories that underpin the teaching process and apply them to teaching practice

■ describe the different domains of learning

■ discuss the factors that will affect the process of learning

■ discuss one of the key supporting structures for learning in practice, namely preceptorship.

ACTIVITY 5.1

Definitions of teaching and learning have been offered elsewhere in this book. It may be helpful to you at this stage to re-read the relevant section in Chapter 1 before we progress with the theories underpinning them.

Dealing solely in definitions is sometimes problematic as it implies that teaching and learning are inseparable. In reality, it is quite possible for learning to take place without any noticeable teaching having occurred.

ACTIVITY 5.2

Try to identify some instances, either in your personal life or in the clinical area, in which you have learned without being actively taught.

There are many examples you may have chosen. In childhood, a great deal of our learning is acquired by experiencing what is happening around us. In the clinical area, many skills, for example, the care of bereaved relatives, are learned by observation and participation.

Having said this, you will probably have noticed that providing definitions of both teaching and learning that are totally independent of each other is practically impossible. Certainly, for this chapter, it is sufficient for us to accept that if a student is to learn, teaching in some guise is likely to have taken place, and if a teacher is to teach, there must be a student to learn. As a result, throughout this and the following chapter, the words 'teaching' and 'learning' will often be used interchangeably.

How we learn is crucial to the whole teaching and learning process, so it is important that this book outlines some of the key thinking that underpins this.

ACTIVITY 5.3

Drawing on your previous experiences as a student, consider what factors ensured that learning had taken place for you.

Your answer may have taken many different directions. For example, you might have included:

- how interesting the subject was
- how approachable the teacher was
- the style adopted by the teacher
- being treated as an adult.

All of these are highly relevant in helping you to learn, and you will have identified many different factors, depending on your own preferences, during the learning process.

THE ADULT LEARNER

Traditionally, most pre- and postregistration courses have been clearly structured, in terms of both the subjects to be learned and how they were to be taught. Changes in thinking in relation to learning styles and developments in new ways of learning, for example, open and distance learning, have led to different approaches being used.

Also, the increase in project or self-directed work now undertaken by students completing their secondary education has led to their having different expectations about how they should be taught. As a result, the expectations of how an individual will be taught depend on his personal experiences.

ACTIVITY 5.4

Think about a programme of study you have recently undertaken. Did you feel that you were treated as an adult? What made you feel this way?

Your views can probably be identified under two headings, as in Box 5.1.

BOX 5.1	*Teaching style*
Not adult centred	*Adult centred*
Formal	Flexible
'Chalk and talk'	Recognises the individual
Teacher decided what was to be learned	Takes account of learning styles
	Student more in control of learning
Timetabled sessions	Large element of discussion
Little or no discussion	Degree of negotiation
No acknowledgement of learning styles	Element of choice

One of the biggest difficulties with other people being in control of our learning is the fact that we do not own it. As a result of this, we view other people as being responsible for it. Ownership of learning is fundamental to the principles of lifelong learning discussed in Chapter 4.

It is important that, as a practitioner, you are aware of the role you have in enabling and supporting students to take responsibility for their own learning.

THE IMPORTANCE OF INDIVIDUAL DIFFERENCES

Ewan and White (1996) highlight the importance of getting to know students' individual characteristics and needs if learning is to be effective. This is largely a result of the individual's own learning style, and is sometimes termed cognitive style.

Research undertaken by psychologists has identified basic differences in our preferred way of learning (Hudson, 1968; Pask, 1976). Put simply, there are many different ways in how we approach and process information. For example, some students find the use of diagrams helpful when learning new information, while others prefer to rely solely on the written word.

Honey and Mumford (cited in Stengelhofen, 1996, pp. 54–55) identify four distinct learning styles that are useful in helping us to understand individual learning needs. They state that the students can be categorised into **activists**, **pragmatists**, **theorists** or **reflectors**. Honey and Mumford devised a questionnaire from which the student can identify his own learning style. A very clear summary of this is given in Stengelhofen (1996, pp. 54–55).

ACTIVITY 5.5

What characteristics do you think individuals would possess in each of the four categories?

The names that have been given to the four categories provide us with a very good indication of the preferred learning style of the individual:

- *Activists*: energetic, easily bored, open minded, enjoy working alongside others.
- *Pragmatists*: dictated by practical consequences rather than theory, like things to happen quickly, receptive to new ideas.
- *Theorists*: systematic, analyse situations, have the ability to reason.
- *Reflectors*: like time to think, thorough, avoid reaching speedy conclusions.

ACTIVITY 5.6

Think where your own learning style might lie in relation to the four categories.

Although the above list provides only a short description, it is clear that the teaching method we use could affect whether a student will learn new information. For example, a student who has an activist learning style may have difficulty learning from a lecture in which there is no student interaction. A reflector may find learning from role play problematic as it depends on an immediate response from the student. Varying your teaching methods will undoubtedly appeal to your students' different learning styles. These are discussed in Chapter 6.

LEARNING THEORIES

Behaviourist theories

These theories are based on what is termed **stimulus – response**. Loosely applied to the teaching situation, this means that the student responds largely to a stimulus, that is, information provided by the teacher, rather than any other forces. This implies that the student is quite passive in the learning process, and learning is largely dependent on input from others. The emphasis is on the 'conditioning' of the student to respond to given situations.

Classical conditioning

The theory of classical conditioning was first described by Pavlov (cited in Curzon, 1985, pp. 19–21), who observed the normal behaviour of dogs. From this, he observed that dogs salivated at the sight of food. This he termed an unconditioned response as it was inherent in the dog without any training being required. In order to develop the experiment further, Pavlov then sounded a bell before the dog received its food and discovered it was possible to train the dog to salivate on the ringing of the bell rather than on the production of the food.

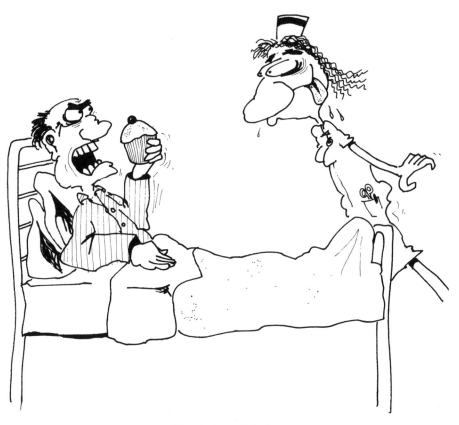

Classical conditioning

Operant conditioning

This theory also relates to stimulus–response but is based on a system of effective training by using rewards. For example, the psychologist Skinner (1968) discovered that it was possible for pigeons to learn how to operate a lever to deliver their food, the food being the reward, or the factor that reinforced their learning of how to use the lever. He used a 'schedule of re-enforcements', which required a consistent approach.

At this juncture, it is quite possible that you are asking how such theory can possibly help you, as a practitioner involved in teaching. This is not necessarily a wrong assumption and is largely supported by Curzon (1985, p. 39), who states that Skinner's 'generalisations concerning human behaviour have been attacked as reflecting the study of animals which are totally unlike human beings. The shaped behaviour of a pigeon taught to dance has been held to be irrelevant to an explanation of the complex activities which form human behaviour.'

ACTIVITY 5.7

Take a few moments to reflect on the above theories. Do you think that you could use them when planning and delivering your teaching? If so, how?

There is a school of thought which reasons that, while acknowledging the need for refinement, Pavlov's work can be used to shape the **intellectual development** of our students The view, much simplified, is based on the fact that as his work is dependent on interaction and surrounding circumstances, it must influence the learning environment. For example, students may learn the type of behaviour expected of them in the classroom situation just by being there.

Cognitive or humanistic learning theories

These theories are more student centred and are, as a result, much easier to apply to our own practice. First, however, it is necessary to identify what is meant by the term **cognition**.

A clear and straightforward definition is the act of knowing, given in the *Concise Oxford Dictionary* (1983). This involves the students' own thinking and **perception**. The approach centres on the work of Carl Rogers (1969). Rogers includes in the act of knowing, the feelings of the student and the need to recognise his individuality.

Constructivist view of learning

This is an extension of the cognitive/humanistic theories of learning. Importance is placed on self-awareness and the individual's understanding of the processes involved in his own learning.

The different views of learning theories are clearly discussed by Kiger (1995, p. 72) who also, in diagrammatic form, neatly categorises the types of theory we need to consider.

Domains of learning

Bloom (1972) has identified three areas or **domains** in which learning takes place, which provide a useful framework for the practitioner involved in teaching. They are identified as:

- The *cognitive* domain, concerned with the acquisition of knowledge.
- The *psychomotor* domain, relating to the development of skills.
- The *affective* domain, involving attitude formation.

The cognitive domain is concerned with how we acquire information and what we need to know as opposed to what we need to do. For example, this could be the effects of compression bandaging on a limb or how insulin works.

The psychomotor domain involves the act of doing or skills acquisition. This could be learning how to give an intramuscular injection or interpret an electro-cardiogram.

The affective domain relates to the development of beliefs, values and attitudes. An example of this is the acceptance of a patient's right to refuse or comply with specific treatment.

The scenario in Box 5.2 will help in your understanding of the three domains.

BOX 5.2   *The three domains of learning*

Sister Bell is teaching compression bandaging to a group of students.

First, she provides the students with knowledge of the circulatory system and how to identify a venous leg ulcer. This is learning in the cognitive domain.

Second, Sister Bell teaches the students how to apply compression bandaging. This lies in the psychomotor domain.

Third, she discusses, with the student, the patient's attitudes to wearing compression bandaging and the need to foster the right attitude if treatment is to be effective. This is learning in the affective domain.

The domains described, known as Bloom's taxonomy, 'may assist the teacher in asking the fundamental questions: In what ways should my students have changed as the result of my teaching and what evidence for the change will I accept?' (Curzon, 1985, p. 107).

ACTIVITY 5.8

Try to identify an aspect of learning that you have recently undertaken. In which of the domains did learning take place?

It is essential to consider all three domains in our teaching even though we may not always use them all.

Relevance to the practitioner as teacher

Beard and Hartley (1984) suggest that no single theory can account for all aspects of learning. However, it would appear that the cognitive theories previously outlined can help students to acquire the problem-solving skills that they will require in their future role.

The stimulus–response or conditioning theories, with their emphasis on rein-forcement, point to the importance of immediate feedback in the learning situation.

CREATING A GOOD LEARNING ENVIRONMENT

The learning environment refers to wherever students are taught. However, Fretwell (1980) and Alexander (1983) have demonstrated that the ward situation is a particularly rich environment for learning, in that students' **motivation** to learn is high during their practical experience (see below). This would seem to confirm that, in nursing, the place where students are most likely to be receptive to teaching and learning is the practice setting. This makes it important that practitioners involved in teaching know how to create an environment that is conducive to learning.

ACTIVITY 5.9

What key elements do you think are essential in creating a good learning environment for your students? To what extent do these aspects exist in your own working environment? If they do not, how can you foster them?

You may have identified the need to be:

- approachable
- welcoming
- confident enough in your work to pass information on to others
- supportive
- helpful
- available and contactable
- knowledgeable.

It is obvious that the more comfortable and safe we feel with the environment, the more likely it is that effective learning will take place.

Some of the aspects you have included in your answer will be developed further below.

MOTIVATION: WHAT MAKES YOU TICK?

To say that a person must wish to learn in order for learning to take place seems self-evident, but there are many factors, within both the teaching and the learning process, that will contribute to the student's wish to learn. Motivation, according to Sargent (1990, p. 4) 'is about what makes people tick'. For example, what makes a student who has completed a diploma course move on to a degree? Or an overworked sister stay on the ward after her span of duty has finished?

Motivation can be described as either **intrinsic** or **extrinsic** to the individual. Intrinsic motivation relates to the personal factors that make us want to learn. The theorist Maslow (1987) provides a good example of intrinsic motivation. He identifies five levels of need that must be met for a person to be 'made to tick'. The five categories of need are as follows:

1. *Physiological.* When applied to student learning, this means that if the student environment is, for example, over– or underheated, noisy, or the student is tired, learning is unlikely to take place or may be limited.

2. *Safety*. This level demonstrates the need to feel safe from danger. For example, students may feel 'unsafe' in an environment where they do not know other students or do not have confidence in the teacher.
3. *Social*. This involves the 'need to be needed' or valued in both our home and working life, for example, to be accepted by our colleagues.
4. *Self-esteem*. When applied to student learning, self-esteem means the need for mutual respect between the individual student, the students as a group and the teacher.
5. *Self-actualisation*. Maslow claims that it is only when these individual needs have been met that the student is able to reach full potential and have the opportunity of 'becoming everything one is capable of becoming' (Sargent, 1990, p. 5).

There are, however, other intrinsic factors that will influence learning, for example, your personal feelings regarding your relationship with other students and teachers.

Extrinsic motivation is that which occurs outside the student and over which he may or may not have control. It is important to note here that the two types of motivation are rarely exclusive of each other. For example, the way in which students are welcomed on to the ward or clinic will affect how they feel (Ogier, 1986).

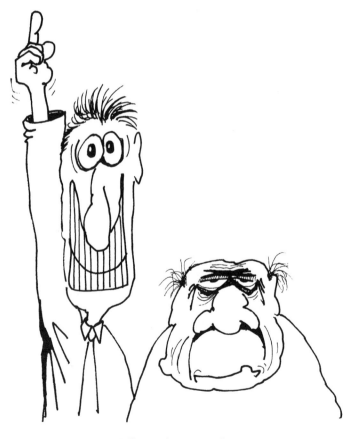

What makes you tick?

ACTIVITY 5.10

Think of a course of study you have recently undertaken. Try to identify the factors that made you want to learn. Were these intrinsic, extrinsic or both?

If the course of study you identified was a course in nursing, it is likely that you identified some of the extrinsic factors of motivation, for example, the need to pass examinations in order to practice in a particular role. Your salary or promotion may depend on it.

Ewan and White (1996) argue that these two aspects are by no means exclusive of each other as students of nursing normally enter the education process with a high degree of intrinsic motivation. This can then be overtaken by extrinsic factors, particularly the need to pass examinations. They go on to say that this is the reason why, in teaching, some students 'are only interested in what they will be asked in the exams' (p. 45).

ACTIVITY 5.11

Having read the section on motivation, take some time to think how you can act as a motivator to the students you work with in the practice setting.

SOCIOLOGICAL FACTORS AFFECTING LEARNING

The most relevant sociological factors that may influence the learning process are those of **language**, **social class** and **culture**.

Bernstein (1962) has identified what he terms a 'restricted language code', which is closely linked to child-rearing practices and education. He argues that people from a working-class background use a limited vocabulary compared with the middle and upper classes, who have a much more elaborate language code. This ultimately affects the way in which people think and make sense of the world around them. If this view is accepted, it would obviously have a bearing on the learning process as teachers and students would not necessarily be 'speaking the same language'.

Another important aspect of language is that of meaning. This is neatly summed up in the phrase 'I know you think you heard what I said, but what I said is not what I meant!' Put another way, the words we sometimes use may contain a different meaning for the person with whom we are communicating. The words of the hospital 'spokesperson' provides us with a perfect example of this: the patient's condition is usually described as 'comfortable' even if the patient is suffering from multiple fractures.

Culture, in its broadest terms, relates to the shared beliefs, values and understanding that are subscribed to by identifying with a particular group. Any student group will link into a culture or **subculture** of one type or another. For example, taking patients or clients as a group, they tend to identify with one another in terms of common problems, and we encourage this by introducing them to self-help groups. The teacher needs to understand the accepted values, attitude and behaviour of the culture or subculture in order to establish a rapport with the student. Mead (1934) states that we all start off by learning roles from our parents and then complete our socialisation by internalising, that is, accepting as our own, the norms and values of other membership groups, at both the cultural and subcultural levels. We also tend to become labelled by others according to the cultures and subcultures in which we find ourselves.

The influences brought to bear culturally on students are of enormous consequence since they may be of far greater importance to the student than those imparted by the teacher. For example, their relationship to their **peer group** is very important to adolescents, and they would often rather please their peers than their family or teachers. As a result, much of what the teacher tries to achieve will be of no consequence if it is not accepted by the peer group.

For example, if you were teaching health promotion to a group of students, you would need to estimate the influence of their peer group. If your session were on the effects of smoking, it would be easier to demonstrate the ill-effects to a group whose peer group did not smoke and whose original socialisation to non-smoking behaviour was because their parents did not smoke. It would obviously be harder to convince a group of the ill-effects of smoking if their parents had always smoked and members of their peer group also did. Teachers must, therefore, be aware that culture can have a great bearing on the effectiveness of learning.

PRECEPTORSHIP: THE ROLE OF THE PRACTITIONER

Preceptorship, as a means of offering support in practice, was outlined in Chapter 1. The purpose of this section is to provide you with the opportunity to reflect on your responsibilities and the skills you will need in order to carry out your role. Preceptorship has been developed in order to help newly registered practitioners to do this.

The UKCC (1995) has stated that all of the newly appointed practitioners 'should be provided with a period of support, where possible under the guidance of a preceptor, for approximately the first four months of registered practice'.

ACTIVITY 5.12

Reflect on your experiences as a newly registered nurse or as a student on the first day of a clinical placement. What level of support did you receive? Was it adequate?

Support in the clinical area has frequently been a somewhat hit-and-miss affair, the level of support depending on pressures of work and staff availability.

ACTIVITY 5.13

What skills do you think you will need in order to act as an effective preceptor to a newly registered nurse? Make a list of the aspects you feel are important. If you are currently a student, what support would you like your preceptor to give you?

In answer to the first question, you will probably have identified on your list aspects such as good communication skills, a professional attitude to your work, a sound knowledge of the area in which you are working and experience in patient/client care. You would also probably expect a preceptor to be a good listener and sympathetic to your anxieties and concerns.

The UKCC also states that preceptors should fulfil the criteria outlined in Box 5.3.

BOX 5.3	*The UKCC's criteria for preceptors*
	■ Be first-level nurses, midwives or health visitors who have normally had at least 12 months' experience within the same or associated clinical fields as the practitioner requiring support ■ Be supporters for the newly registered practitioner, a colleague who can act as a valuable source of help, both professionally and personally, during the early months of registered practice ■ Negotiate the nature of the role and relationship with the practitioner concerned ■ Recognise that newly registered practitioners are accountable for their own actions, as set out in the UKCC *Code of Professional Conduct* (1992b)

Preceptorship is not a legal requirement in nursing, but it is a clear example of what is termed 'good practice' by providing a high level of support at the start of the practitioner's career or on re-entering registered practice following a career break. In view of this, there is no formal training for preceptors, and this responsibility is usually assumed by employers. Before becoming preceptors, practitioners should discuss the following aspects with their manager.

The outcomes of the preparation should be that you, as a preceptor, will:

■ have sufficient understanding of educational programmes leading to registration to be able to identify ongoing learning needs
■ be able to assist the newly registered practitioner to apply theory to practice
■ have an understanding of the issues involved in integrating the practitioner into the practice setting
■ support the practitioner in the transition from preregistration student status to that of a registered and accountable practitioner
■ foster professional development.

CONCLUSION

This chapter has focused on the factors that are likely to have a bearing on the ways in which we learn and how we can maximise learning in our own working environment. The fact that teaching and learning are closely linked will also influence the way in which we teach, in either the classroom or the practice setting. The next chapter will provide you with the framework within which to develop your teaching skills while, at the same time, maximising learning in the students with whom you are working.

GLOSSARY

Activist: a person who directs energy towards a political goal.

Cognition: a term given to the internal mental processes such as perceiving, learning, thinking and problem-solving.

Culture: the customs and rules of a particular group of people based on a shared belief system, including accepted ways of living one's life.

Domain: sphere, province or scope.

Extrinsic: external to the individual or organism.

Intellectual development: the development of the faculty of knowing and reasoning.

Intrinsic: within or internal to the individual or organism.

Language: the code by which human beings communicate.

Motivation: that which impels a person to action.

Peer group: a group of people who are associated and of equal status, usually sharing a common approach such as dress, language, values and recreation.

Pragmatist: a person concerned with practical consequences or values.

Reflector: a person who thinks through and draws off previous experience before reaching a decision or viewpoint.

Social class: formally, the method by which the population is categorised, usually by employment. Also implies certain types of behaviour and culture.

Stimulus – response: a view that all behaviour occurs in response to stimuli.

Sub-culture: a group within a culture sharing the same patterns of beliefs, behaviour, attitudes and values, which are distinguishable from the overall culture of the society.

Taxonomy: a structure that describes different aspects of the learning process.

Theorist: word usually used in relation to practice in nursing. Involves thought, ideas and reasoning.

REFERENCES

Alexander MF (1983) *Learning to Nurse: Integrating Theory and Practice.* Edinburgh: Churchill Livingstone.

Beard RM and Hartley J (1984) *Teaching in Higher Education*, 4th edn. London: Harper & Row.

Bernstein B (1962) Linguistic codes, hesitation phenomena and intelligence. *Language and Speech*, 5 (Jan–Mar), 15–17.

Bloom BS (1972) *Taxonomy of Educational Objectives*, London: Longman.

Concise Oxford Dictionary (1983) Oxford: Oxford University Press.

Curzon LB (1985) *Teaching in Further Education: An Outline of Principles and Practice*, 3rd edn. Eastbourne: Holt, Rinehart & Winston.

Ewan C and White R (1996) *Teaching Nursing: A Self Instructional Handbook*, 2nd edn. London: Chapman & Hall.

Fretwell JE (1980) An enquiry into the ward learning environment. *Nursing Times Occasional Paper*, 6(20), 69–75.

Hudson L (1968) *Frames of Mind. Ability, Perception and Self Perception in the Arts and Sciences.* London: Methuen.

Kiger AM (1995) *Teaching for Health*, 2nd edn. New York: Churchill Livingstone.

Maslow AH (1987) *Motivation and Personality*, London: Harper & Row.

Mead GH (1934) *Mind, Self and Society.* Chicago: University of Chicago Press.

Ogier ME (1986) An ideal sister – seven years on. *Nursing Times Occasional Paper*, 82(2): 54–57.

Pask G (1976) Styles and strategies of learning. *British Journal of Educational Psychology*, 46, 128–148.

Rogers C (1969) *Freedom to Learn.* Columbus, OH: Charles E. Merrill.

Sargent A (1990) *Turning People on: The*

Motivation Challenge. London: Institute of Personnel Management.

Skinner BF (1968) *The Technology of Teaching.* New York: Appleton-Century-Croft.

Stengelhofen J (1996) *Teaching Students in Clinical Settings.* London: Chapman & Hall.

United Kingdom Central Council for Nursing, Midwifery and Health Visiting (1992a) *The Scope of Professional Practice,* London: UKCC.

United Kingdom Central Council for Nursing, Midwifery and Health Visiting (1992b) *Code of Professional Conduct for Nurses, Midwives and Health Visitors.* London: UKCC.

United Kingdom Central Council for Nursing, Midwifery and Health Visiting (1995) *The Council's Position Concerning a Period of Support for Nurses, Midwives and Health Visitors Entering or Re-entering Registered Practice.* Registrar's letter 3/1995. London: UKCC.

FURTHER READING

Cole P and Chan L (1994) *Teaching Principles and Practice,* 2nd edn. Australia: Prentice Hall. *This is a very useful textbook that identifies appropriate models for teaching in addition to helpful information on its planning and preparation.*

Ewan C and White R (1996) *Teaching Nursing: A Self Instructional Handbook,* 2nd edn. London: Chapman & Hall. *This book further develops the aspects of learning outlined in this chapter. It is particularly useful if you are preparing work in isolation as it contains many useful exercises to check your understanding of the learning process.*

Kiger A (1995) *Teaching For Health,* 2nd edn. New York: Churchill Livingstone. *While this book is largely related to teaching health promotion, it provides a very useful chapter on the various learning theories, some of which are presented in a very clear diagrammatic form.*

Sotto E (1994) *When Teaching Becomes Learning. Theory and Practice of Teaching.* London: Cassell Education. *This book contains a very useful chapter on the learning process and develops the different approaches to learning already outlined in this book.*

6 Strategies for meeting learning needs

Sue Howard

INTRODUCTION

Even the most confident and competent of teachers will admit to a degree of nervousness when asked to undertake a presentation for the first time, but with the right approach and preparation, this can become a very enjoyable part of the practitioner's role. The purpose of this chapter is, therefore, to provide you with the 'how to' of teaching by giving you a framework within which to make your teaching effective. It will identify strategies that you can employ in order to maximise the learning in your students and enable you to plan your teaching appropriately.

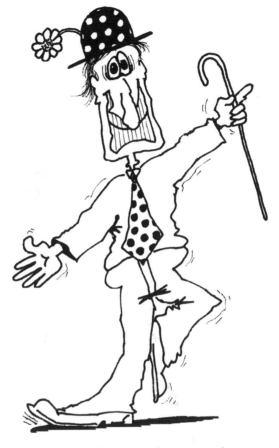

Strategies for meeting learning needs

LEARNING OBJECTIVES

After reading this chapter, you should be able to:

- recognise the value of reflective practice in developing a teaching strategy
- discuss the role of the practitioner in supporting learning needs in both formal and informal settings
- select the most appropriate teaching method based on learning need
- complete a formal teaching plan based on specific objectives
- evaluate the effectiveness of your teaching.

BUILDING THE FRAMEWORK: WHY WE NEED A TEACHING STRATEGY

A strategy, in its simplest form, is concerned with forward planning. The *Concise Oxford Dictionary* (1983) describes it as 'the art of war; especially the part of it concerned with the conduct of campaigns'. This may appear to be a rather extreme definition, but for those of you who have had the experience of teaching a group of over 250 preregistration diploma students, it is unlikely that you would deny the need to be organised. What is also apparent is that, as individuals, we all have different concerns and worries regarding our teaching and how it is received.

Jolly (1997) suggests that the transition from a student teacher to a qualified teacher in the classroom situation is problematic, particularly in relation to integration. This is largely brought about because the teacher has not yet developed a sense of belonging in relation to the educational establishment concerned. Clifford (1995) also cites conflicts and challenges for nurse teachers as they attempt to meet the diverse aspects of their role. It could be argued that this is equally applicable to practitioners who are asked to teach in similar circumstances. As a practitioner and as a teacher, then, the starting point is one of survival.

THE VALUE OF REFLECTIVE PRACTICE

You will already have identified from the earlier chapters the value of reflective practice to the teacher and to the whole of the learning process. The principles of this are particularly relevant to this chapter, both in terms of enhancing the learning experience for the student and in helping you, as a practitioner and a teacher, to develop your teaching skills (see also Chapter 4).

ACTIVITY 6.1

Using the knowledge you have gained from Chapter 4, consider how adopting reflective practice and maintaining a reflective journal will assist in your understanding of this chapter.

You will have learned that reflection is about analysing a situation in order to decide on the best way forward and to learn from it. Boud et al (1985) identify a preparatory phase in the reflective process in which the student consciously anticipates the experience. It is argued that this is an essential part of learning and that its value should not be overlooked. In view of this, reflection is concerned with looking forward to experiences as well as learning from what has passed.

Shields (1994, p. 755) identifies four key points that are crucial to becoming proficient in the process of reflective practice:

- the need for conscious and voluntary effort
- its usefulness as a tool in helping you to explore the links between what you are told and your observations in practice
- the importance of journal writing in assisting the reflective process
- the need to work through initial difficulties in journal writing as these diminish with persistence and practice.

The importance of journal, log or diary writing to learning

These have become a popular method of learning, particularly when the learning is self-directed. They provide a very useful tool from which to explore beliefs and values in terms of your own experiences. Journals can also provide a very powerful teaching tool when used as the basis for group discussion or in one-to-one tutorials. This aspect will be discussed in greater depth later in this chapter.

The main aim of a journal is to help you or your student to develop skills of reflection, evaluation and decision-making. However, probably the most important aspect for you, as a practitioner, is its place in helping to forge the links between theory and practice. In view of this, before we look at how to write a journal, it is useful to look at the relationship between theory and practice.

LINKING THEORY WITH PRACTICE: THE ROLE OF THE PRACTITIONER

As a practitioner, you are likely to be aware of the term 'theory–practice gap'. The fundamental mistake we make is that we see it as a new problem brought about by changes in both the education and practice of nursing. In reality, it is not a new concept, and as long as 50 years ago, the need for the integration of theory and practice was highlighted (Balme, 1937; cited in Alexander, 1982, p. 65).

In addition, there are many different perceptions of what has become termed the theory–practice gap, making the issue extremely complex (McCaugherty, 1992). Before we look at your role in bridging it, it is essential to identify what you, as a practitioner, perceive to be a theory – practice gap.

ACTIVITY 6.2

Think about your current role. Do you believe there to be a gap in the application of practice to theory? Why do you think this is?

The aspects you have identified will depend on your current role and will probably include one or more of the following:

- theory being purely 'academic', for example, where it is not seen in practice
- nursing students not being able to transfer what they have learned in the classroom to the practical situation
- a lack of contact with the teachers providing the theory
- a lack of information from the institution providing the theory.

Although the reasons for the theory – practice gap are diverse, there are many ways in which you, as a practitioner, can close it. These are by gaining an understanding of the curriculum and processes in operation where these impact on you in your work (see the section on the curriculum, below).

ACTIVITY 6.3

If learning is to take place, it is crucial that you are able to assist the student to apply the theory that she has learned in the classroom to her area of practice. Take some time to consider how you might do this.

You have probably included in your answer aspects such as having an understanding of what students are being taught in theory, your own attitudes and beliefs, the time available, levels of motivation, etc. From this, it is clear that journal-writing is only one way in which we can build links between theory and practice.

HOW TO WRITE A JOURNAL, LOG OR DIARY OF LEARNING

One of the key aspects that must be stressed in relation to personal journals is that of confidentiality. This is implicit in the United Kingdom Central Council for Nursing, Midwifery and Health Visiting (UKCC) *Code of Professional Conduct* (1992). No material written in the journal should make it possible to identify any patient or client by either name or inference.

Dewing (1990) identifies some useful ground rules if personal journals are to form the basis of group discussion:

1. The journal is the property of the nurse who writes it.
2. Writers are free to reveal as much or as little of the content of their journal as they wish.
3. Shared information is not to be revealed to others without consent.
4. Comments on other nurses' reflections must be positive and supportive.
5. Nurses commenting on each others' reflections must work together as a peer group.

With the increased emphasis on reflective practice as a valuable contributor to the teaching process, it is natural to assume that it is a relatively new concept. However, probably the most straightforward definition of a journal as a reflective tool was provided by Baldwin (1977, p. 10), who differentiated between a journal and a diary by describing a diary as a record of observations and experiences, and a journal as a 'tool for recording the process of our lives'.

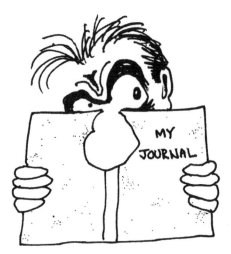

Writing a journal

Generally speaking, diaries are much more superficial and are used for recording day-to-day events. Journals may not only contain experiences and activities, but also incorporate the writer's reflections and the impact that these have on her life. Prognoff (1975) argues that maintaining a journal provides continuity for the student by enabling her to reflect on specific events and periods, record them and then carry out a dialogue, linking past and present events and reactions to them. Journals can be very helpful during times of change brought about by circumstances external to the writer. Reviewing how one handled previous changes may offer strategies for how to handle the present situation.

Writing thoughts and feelings may be cathartic in itself. Prognoff (1975) found that reading aloud made a stronger impact on the reader than did silent reading. Journals also have the advantage of allowing the writer to return to past entries and re-read them in order to gain some insight into the present.

Recording your journal

How you actually record is a matter of personal choice. Loose-leaf notebooks provide much greater flexibility as pages can be added and removed when required. Whatever its format, the journal should be used solely for the purpose of recording your journal entries; that is, it should not be used, for example, to jot down telephone messages or patient notes. Some practical tips on keeping a journal are outlined in Box 6.1.

BOX 6.1	*Practical tips for keeping a journal*
	<ul><li>Remember that the main aim of the journal is your own self-development.</li><li>It is not as much work as it appears. The more you use it the easier it becomes.</li><li>Try to write entries at least once or twice a week.</li><li>Be brief. Only write as much as necessary to get your point across, but avoid just making lists.</li><li>Try to focus on the *now* in your life or the very recent past, that is, the past few days.</li><li>Make at least one positive statement about yourself, your strengths or your abilities in each entry.</li><li>Review your entry every month and rewrite all the positive comments you have made about yourself during that time.</li><li>Your journal is private to you so you can be totally honest with yourself.</li><li>Do not analyse too much by re-reading your entries. You will get the feedback you need to help you to develop by discussion.</li><li>Take great care to ensure that the patient/client is not identifiable. The journal is private to you, but we are all human and things do get mislaid.</li></ul>

The implementation in 1995 of the UKCC's postregistration education and practice (PREP) requirements has led to an increase in the use of reflective diaries as a means of demonstrating how learning has influenced patient/client care. This has, in turn, led to concern regarding who should have access to the information contained within it. For example, in the unlikely event of the patient or client discussed in the journal or diary being the focus of court proceedings, could the contents be used as evidence? To date, there are no known instances of this occurring so it is difficult to forecast its possibility. However, while there is even the slightest possibility that portfolio entries could be relevant in litigation, it is absolutely crucial that it is not possible to recognise any patient or client in your journal. Taking time to think how you are going to achieve this is an integral part of maintaining your journal or diary. In addition, a useful tip at the end of each entry is to ask yourself the fundamental question 'Would anyone be able to identify the patient or client from what I have written?' If this is the case, it must be reworded.

An excellent introduction to reflective journals is provided by Ghaye (1996).

FORMAL AND INFORMAL TEACHING

Teaching is often described as being either formal or informal. Formal refers to the type of teaching that is preplanned, often with a clear aim and objectives. Informal teaching refers to the spontaneous type of teaching that occurs when a situation presents itself.

ACTIVITY 6.4

Think about your current role. Which aspects of your work do you think would be best taught (a) formally, and (b) informally?

Under the formal heading, you may have included aspects such as the safe moving and handling of patients or the care of essential equipment. Informal teaching could include the changing of intravenous fluids, which the student can observe at the bedside. Both types of teaching have advantages and disadvantages.

ACTIVITY 6.5

Make a list of the advantages and disadvantages of each method of teaching.

The major advantages of using a formal method are that usually both the student and teacher know exactly what the session aims to achieve and it enables the student to undertake her own preparation, for example, by selecting some background reading. The major advantages of using an informal method are that it is meaningful for the student and helps to ensure that the knowledge she is gaining is up to date. This is often regarded as a form of **action learning**.

The teaching of nursing as a subject usually occurs by a combination of the two methods.

DECIDING WHAT TO TEACH

It is obvious that, in nurse education programmes, decisions have to be taken about what the students should learn. Abbatt and McMahon (1993, p. 17) put this in a nutshell.

> If there is a course for orthopaedic surgeons it should be totally different from a course for health inspectors. Health inspectors do not need to be able to replace hip joints and orthopaedic surgeons do not need to control the breeding sites of mosquitoes.

In the same way, nurse education programmes need to be relevant to the area of work that students will be expected to undertake on completion of the course. This is achieved by curriculum planning and the selection of an appropriate **curriculum model** with which to design the course.

Many of you reading this chapter will be familiar with using nursing models in order to plan and prioritise care. In the same way, formalised programmes of nurse education are based on curriculum models. A curriculum model, as defined by Burrel (1988), refers to the organised setting out of the key elements of what should be learned, either using the written word or in diagrammatic form.

This section will provide you with only a brief introduction to curriculum models. For those of you requiring a more in-depth knowledge, an excellent outline of curriculum planning and **curriculum design** is given in Quinn (1994).

The *product model* of curriculum design is based on the 'end result' of education (usually an award or qualification) and the need to meet specific objectives. Learning is seen as a change in observable behaviour and is measured against the students' achievement of the objectives.

The *process model* of curriculum design is concerned with the progression of learning as being of benefit in itself as opposed to in terms of outcome. Therefore, students are allowed to develop at their own pace, there are no set objectives and, as a result, what is learned may be unpredictable.

ACTIVITY 6.6

What do you think would be the benefits of each of the two models when teaching in your own area of practice?

The use of a product model in some aspects of nurse teaching is extremely useful, especially when the completion of an end product of learning, for example, the teaching of fire evacuation procedures to a new student on the ward, is required.

The process model is much more focused on the development of understanding and requires a more active role from the students. It allows them to develop the skills they need at their own pace. The teacher in this model acts as a **facilitator**, supporting rather than 'telling' the student what to do. There are no set outcomes to achieve by a given time. For example, the student learns over time how to prioritise care.

As a practitioner, facilitator or teacher, it is important that you are familiar with the curriculum design of the courses with which you are involved. The following is a useful list of questions to ask when in discussion with a relevant lecturer–practitioner:

1. What is the **philosophy** on which the curriculum is based?
2. Which curriculum model has been chosen and why?
3. How do the different parts fit together to provide an overall package for the students? For example, how are the students able to relate theory to practice and vice versa?
4. How is progression demonstrated throughout the curriculum?
5. Does the curriculum allow for differences in learning style?
6. Does the curriculum allow for different teaching methods?
7. How is the curriculum assessed?
8. Does the model allow the student to take responsibility for her own learning?

DIFFERENT APPROACHES TO TEACHING

As stated in Chapter 5, the terms 'teaching' and 'learning' are often used interchangeably. It is, therefore, appropriate to explore some additional theories that are helpful to our understanding of the teaching process.

Androgogy and pedagogy

The successful teacher is no longer on a height, pumping knowledge at high pressure into passive receptacles ... He is a senior student anxious to help his juniors. (Sir William Osler, 1849–1919)

ACTIVITY 6.7

Apart from the fact that the above quotation is less gender-friendly than we would expect to see today, it is difficult to imagine that this was written so long ago. Reflect on what this statement means to you. How far do you agree with it?

There are two key issues to emerge from the statement. First, effective teaching requires more than just telling someone else what you think they ought to know, and second, the inference is that teaching is helping someone else to learn.

Definitions

Probably the most straightforward definition of androgogy is provided by Knowles (1984), who defines it as 'the art and science of helping adults to learn'. This is contrasted with pedagogy, which means 'the art and science of teaching children'. It is argued that there are fundamental differences in these two approaches that will ultimately affect how students learn. Box 6.2 identifies these differences.

BOX 6.2	*Androgogy and pedagogy*

Androgogy

- Learning occurs as a result of the student's own effort.
- The teacher and students treat each other as equals in the teaching and learning process.
- The teaching methods selected are student centred.
- The students accept responsibility for their own learning.

Pedagogy

- Learning occurs as a result of the input of others.
- The student–teacher partnership is unequal. Students 'look up' to the teacher.
- Teaching methods are teacher led.
- The teacher accepts responsibility for the students' learning.

This idea is further developed by Quinn (1988), who states that teaching can be divided into two broad categories: traditional and progressive. Traditional teaching is characterised by its teacher centredness, with the student assuming a passive role. The progressive approach is much more student orientated, with the student playing an active role.

ACTIVITY 6.8

From the above, it is clear that an androgogical approach to teaching is different as it involves students being treated as adults. Think of your own experiences as a student. What led you to believe you were being treated as an adult as opposed to the teacher having total responsibility?

You will probably have identified some of the following:

1. mutual respect
2. being approachable
3. a willingness to discuss rather than dictate
4. accepting people for what they are
5. accepting their personal values.

Rogers (1983) states that effective teaching refers to a set of features that may characterise a number of different processes:

- It must involve learning and possibly teaching.
- The content of what is taught must be thought valuable.
- The teaching method used must be considered morally acceptable to both the teacher and student.

Rogers also provides us with a very useful framework for practitioners who are also involved in teaching in practice:

1. *The importance of establishing a climate of trust.* This is largely self-explanatory. From our own experiences, we can undoubtedly recognise the needs we have in feeling accepted as a person, secure in the knowledge that we are valued.

2. *Being aware of the individual learning needs of the student.* This involves being aware of the student's current knowledge, for example, the stage of training reached and her competence in undertaking certain procedures.
3. *The importance of student motivation* to the learning process (see Chapter 5).
4. *Exposure to a wide range of experiences.*

Think about the types of experience that are available in your area of work and how you could ensure that the students have access to these.

5. *Acting as a resource.* This means acting as a 'signpost' in order to direct students to the information they may require. For example, you may need to refer to work that is undertaken in another department or highlight available literature.

There are many opportunities in your day-to-day work that can be used as a vehicle for enabling your students to learn. You may, in your earlier list, have identified ward or community reports. The information that is shared and discussed provides an excellent learning opportunity for the student. For the same reasons, ward rounds can be of great value. Taking part in the ward round also has the added benefit of observing multidisciplinary approaches to care and makes the students feel part of the team. Involving students in nursing care/case conferences also reinforces the importance of collabora-tion and cooperation with other organisations in the provision of patient/ client care.

6. *Accepting the student as a person.* While we all try to get along with our colleagues, it is a fact of life that we prefer being with some people rather than others. This is usually because their personalities are compatible with our own. From this, it is likely that at some stage in our careers and despite great effort on both sides, a personality clash is unavoidable. Should this be the case, it is better to discuss this openly with all the parties involved so that the issue can be addressed in the best interest of all concerned.

7. *Sharing the student's thoughts and feelings.* This involves all aspects of 'being there' for the student and sharing feelings in relation to events in the practice situation. It also means making the student feel wanted as a learner. It is important for us, as practitioners, to remember that for every nurse who has been aware of supervising a disinterested student, there is a student who feels that she has had a disinterested facilitator or **mentor**.

8. *Using conflict and tensions as a learning experience.* This means talking through with the student distressing or disturbing experiences that she may have encountered. For example, decisions taken regarding patient resuscita-tion can be extremely upsetting when first encountered by students.

9. *Accepting one's own strengths and weaknesses.* Implicit in this is the need for you, as a facilitator, to accept your own limitations, safe in the knowledge that you cannot know everything there is to know about your area of practice or be all things to all people. Accepting your own strengths and weaknesses requires you to look objectively at yourself and try to improve on some aspects of your role, while at the same time acknowledging that at which you are proficient.

PREPARING YOUR TEACHING

One of the greatest difficulties for most practitioners faced with teaching for the first time is where to start. From reading Chapter 5, it is clear that the teaching method you select may affect the way in which students learn, so an assessment of your student or student group is essential.

ACTIVITY 6.10

Think about your experiences as a student. Which teaching methods did you prefer and why?

Your answer will undoubtedly reflect your personal learning style. There is, however, a sequence of events that can be applied regardless of the method selected. There is an old adage that is well known to teachers:

Tell'em what you're going to tell 'em.
Then tell 'em.
Then tell 'em what you've just told 'em!

This principle can be applied to other situations. Next time you have the opportunity to view one of the old Hollywood-style slapstick comedies with the 'custard pie in the face' routine, watch carefully the sequence of events:

1. The 'deliverer' of the custard pie indicates what is going to happen, i.e. he is going to let the 'receiver' have it in the face! (Tell'em what you're going to tell 'em.)
2. The 'deliverer' delivers said custard pie to the 'recipient'. (Then tell 'em.)
3. The 'deliverer' holds empty plate, indicates the content on 'receiver's' face and laughs. (Tell'em what you've just told 'em!)

The sequence of events when planning teaching is therefore,

- the introduction
- the progression of the subject material
- the conclusion.

The introduction includes 'setting the scene' for the session, finding out what the students already know and telling them why they need to learn the knowledge and the method by which they are to learn it. (In Chapter 5, how the last two points increase learning in the student was discussed.)

Equally as important, regardless of the teaching method you choose, is the way in which you communicate with your students.

COMMUNICATION SKILLS

As we have seen earlier in this chapter, recent years have seen dramatic changes in the way we are taught, moving from a pedagogical to an androgogical approach. Fundamental to this approach is the way in which we communicate our teaching material. The following are some general rules to follow, both in preparation and during your teaching:

- Ask open as opposed to closed questions, for example:

  – What do you understand by that?
  – How would you do this?
  – What other view might you consider?

- Show an understanding of other people's feelings. You may be nervous teaching, but the student may also be afraid to speak.
- Listen carefully to what a student has to say.
- Silence is possibly one of the most difficult situations to deal with when teaching, and 20 seconds' silence when you have posed a question really does seem like a lifetime. This makes you vulnerable to answering your own questions before waiting for the student's response.

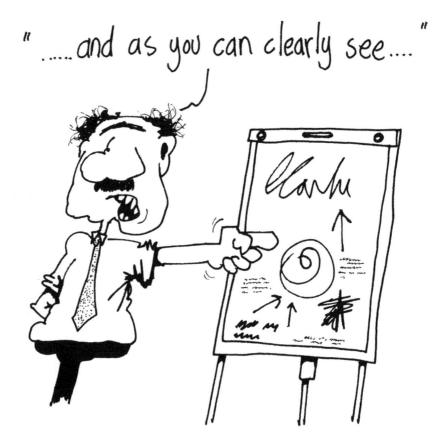

Communication skills

ACTIVITY 6.11

Position yourself as if you were speaking at the front of the class and ask any question. It does not matter what it is. Now wait for 20 seconds. You will soon learn how long this can feel.

- Give students alternatives. There is often more than one way of achieving the same goal.
- Make sure that your facts are correct.
- Do not be afraid of saying that you do not have an answer. Teachers never could, nor should they, know everything.
- Admit it openly if you get something wrong.

The use of humour in teaching

Parkin (1989) argues that, when used properly, humour is one of the most important qualities of a good teacher. There is only one major rule regarding the use of humour in your teaching: it should be appropriate and linked closely with the content of your teaching.

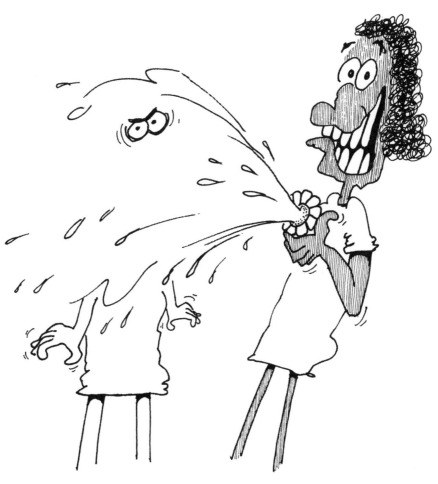

Use of humour

Having looked at some of the general issues, the following is a basic, but none the less useful, framework to use that will help you to feel more confident. It is often termed the 'what, why, when, where and how of teaching'.

The what of teaching

This aspect is not always quite as straightforward as it sounds, and many practitioners make the mistake of overlooking it. For example, you may be asked to deliver a teaching session on the moving and handling of patients, but what aspects of moving and handling are you required to teach? In reality, this can encompass legislation, aids to assist moving and handling, patient safety, nurse safety and employer policy. The possibilities are almost endless. This lesson was brought home to me very early in my teaching career when I was asked to deliver 10 hours' teaching on the learning environment!

Using the following as a guide will assist you in deciding exactly what you want the students to learn:

- First of all, seek a clear answer to the fundamental question of what part of the subject you are being asked to teach. This will not only reduce your stress levels, but also enable you to focus your teaching and ensure that you are not repeating content that has already been taught.
- Having identified the subject matter (you may sometimes have to be quite persistent about this), you are then in a position to develop the aim and specific objectives for the session (see below). While it is acknowledged that the formulation of objectives may not always be the best way to plan your teaching, it does enable you, if you are new to teaching, to be much more focused.

The importance of evidence-based practice

Evidence-based practice has been described as the bridge between research and nursing practice (Curzio, 1997). From this, it is incumbent on the teacher to ensure that her teaching material is from the same evidence base. This can be achieved by always ensuring that you research your subject fully, and by providing the students with the evidence to support your statements and views.

One of the key purposes of evidence-based practice is to ensure that the patient/client receives up-to-date care based on up-to-date knowledge. It is, therefore, vital to the learning process that your information is not based on 'history'. The easiest way of ensuring this is by undertaking a literature search on the subject you are intending to teach. Your college of nursing library will be able to assist you in this. It is important that your search is highly focused on what you want to know. For example, if you entered the words 'nursing process', you would get over 1000 'hits', which is obviously not much help. By asking yourself what exactly it is that you wish to know about the nursing process, you will narrow the subject down drastically, and the information you receive will be much more manageable and pertinent.

The why of teaching

In order for you to gain an understanding of what is required in terms of teaching, it is essential to know why a particular subject is to be taught. For example:

- Is the subject an examinable part of the curriculum?
- If this is the case, what aspects of the subject *must* the students know?
- Does it link with previously taught subjects?

The when of teaching

There are five fundamental questions that you may find useful (Box 6.3).

BOX 6.3	Questions for the 'when' of teaching
	1. How much time have you been allocated for the session? 2. Is the time sufficient for what you have been asked to do? 3. How does what you have been asked to teach fit into the module or course? For example, is it a 'stand-alone' session or one of a series? 4. If others are teaching on the same subject, how can you ensure that there is no overlap or repetition? 5. How will your teaching and the students' learning be evaluated?

The where of teaching

This may appear self-explanatory, but the changing numbers of student groups and the frequent, limited use of classroom accommodation often lead to various annexed buildings being used. It may be that your teaching is to take place in the practice area. If so, you will need to consider exactly where to carry out the teaching in order to avoid any distractions.

The how of teaching

Having gained the above information and established your objectives, you are now in a position to decide what is the most appropriate teaching method for the subject material you are to deliver.

PROVIDING A STRUCTURE FOR TEACHING

Aims and objectives

The development of aims and objectives as a framework for a planned teaching session is extremely useful. First, they provide a logical sequence for both you and your student, and second, they enable you to check whether your teaching has been effective. Central to the development of aims and objectives is the decision about what exactly the student should learn.

Identifying what to teach

This is often described as the must, should and could of teaching, and although it is a simple framework, it will provide you with some very useful pegs on which to hang your subject material.

ACTIVITY 6.12

Think of a subject of which you have a sound knowledge. Here are some examples to help with your choice:

- accidental hypothermia in older people
- the safe storage of drugs
- planning off-duty rotas
- care of a patient immediately following surgery.

Having found your subject, try to identify what you feel the students must know, should know and could know about the subject you have chosen.

To take the safe storage of drugs as an example, you may feel that the students *must* know the following:

- the law relating to drug storage
- your employer's policy on storage
- the process of recording stored drugs.

What they *should* know, that is, desirable additions to the must-knows, are the wider issues involved, for example, the ordering and disposal of stored drugs. Finally, what the students *could* know, that is, non-essential but optional knowledge, is the patient's/client's role in storage.

This can provide a useful framework for identifying what is the most important content of your teaching and so should enable you to formulate its aim.

Identifying your aim for the session

An aim in teaching terms is an overall statement that identifies what the student must be able to do at the end of a given period of instruction or experience.

ACTIVITY 6.13

With this definition in mind, try to formulate an aim for the subject that you identified in 6.12.

There are two key aspects to remember when identifying your aim: first, it is a general statement of what is to be achieved and second, it should state why it is worth achieving.

To use the example previously given of accidental hypothermia in older people, the aim for the teaching would be something like 'At the end of the session, students will understand the nature of accidental hypothermia in older people, in order that they can deliver skilled nursing care.' You will notice that the aim does not tell you *how* this will be achieved. This is done in the next step, by formulating educational objectives or what are now often called (intended) learning outcomes.

Generally speaking, objectives or learning outcomes must:

- be achievable within the period allocated for the teaching
- be specific in terms of what you want the student to achieve
- be measurable in terms of their outcome.

Again, to use the risk of accidental hypothermia in older people as an example, the educational objectives could be as follows:

At the end of the session students should be able to:

- explain the predisposing causes of accidental hypothermia in older people
- recognise the signs and symptoms of accidental hypothermia in this client group
- describe the treatment of a patient suffering from accidental hypothermia
- recognise the factors that make older people more at risk of accidental hypothermia.

As a general rule by which to measure your objectives or learning outcomes, always ask whether they are:

1. Specific
2. Measurable
3. Achievable
4. Realistic
5. Time limited.

As useful as SMART objectives are in helping you to decide what to teach, they do have certain limitations.

ACTIVITY 6.14

Make a list of all the positive and negative aspects of teaching by objectives that you can think of.

The positive aspects may include that they:

- provide your teaching with a clear and logical structure
- enable the teacher to control the timing
- make it easier to ascertain what the student has learned
- provide a clear record of what has been taught
- enable students to direct their own study.

The negative aspects may include that they:

- are time consuming to prepare (although this improves with practice)
- tend to be inflexible
- limit the content of the session and, as a result, what the student will learn.

On balance, if you are new to teaching, using objectives when preparing to teach is invaluable.

There is a wealth of information available to assist you in formulating your educational objectives. You may find the text by Abbatt and McMahon (1993) particularly useful.

TEACHING METHODS

Having identified what it is that you are going to teach, you are then in a position to select an appropriate teaching method. There are many different methods that you can utilise, each of which has its advantages and disadvantages. It is true to say, however, that the method selected needs to correspond to the domain of learning in which it is to take place if the learning is to be effective (see Chapter 4). The lecture method is of little value if you wish to change students' attitudes on a given subject. For example, it is highly unlikely that you would change a student's opinion that inequalities in health care were justifiable by just lecturing to her.

The method chosen will also depend on the number of students you are going to teach, and there may be occasions when because of the large number of students involved, the lecture is the only appropriate method. There are a variety of teaching methods that you can use:

■ lectures
■ group discussions
■ seminars
■ role play
■ learning from critical incidents
■ independent/directed learning
■ experiential learning.

The lecture

The terms 'lecture' and 'lesson' are frequently used interchangeably, although a lesson tends to involve more student interaction. The lecture largely involves the teacher doing most of the talking and the students listening. This is an extremely valuable teaching method when you wish to provide the students with particular knowledge, for example, the functions of the liver or the results of research.

The advantages of using the lecture method are as follows:

■ It is extremely efficient in terms of teacher time as, so far as accommodation allows, the session can be delivered to large numbers of students at the same time.
■ It is a very useful way of introducing new topics.
■ As the topics are new, they may act as a motivator for the students.
■ The knowledge you provide can be totally up to date.
■ It provides a useful framework on which to base other sessions. For example, the students may all be given the same information and, at a later date, formed into groups to discuss it.

Some of the criticisms levelled at the lecture method are at best derogatory. WH Auden, cited in Curzon (1985, p. 191), states that 'the lecturer is a person who talks in someone else's sleep', which might at first glance be a bit offputting to the new lecturer, but should instill in us the need to make the subject we are going to teach of interest. Some other criticisms of the lecture method are:

■ The students are mainly passive. (The students may see this as a plus!)
■ It may not appeal to the student's individual learning style.
■ The opportunity to explore the issues raised is limited.
■ It is difficult for the teacher to ascertain whether she has been understood.

Handouts

Handouts are a very useful tool from which the students can have a record of what you have taught during the lecture. They also have the added advantage of enabling the student to concentrate on what you are saying rather than taking notes. Whether or not you use them, however, will depend on the time you have in which to prepare them and the facilities you have available to produce them. There are two basic types: the handout on which you provide all the key points of your lecture, and the 'gapped' handout, which gives the student the main headings and space between each one to enable her to complete it during the lecture.

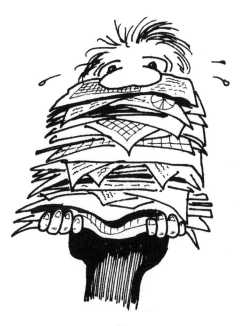

Handouts

There are five key areas that you should include on a handout:

1. the topic being taught
2. the aim and objectives (or learning outcome) of the session
3. a statement of the main points of the presentation
4. a summary of the main points
5. an up-to-date list of further reading that students can access if they require more information.

If you were to present a lecture on the effects of smoking on health, a gapped handout would look something like that in Box 6.4. The student then completes the handout from the information given during the lecture.

BOX 6.4	*An example of a lecture handout*

1. *Title*: The Effects of Smoking on Health
2. *Learning outcomes*: At the end of the session, students should be able to:
   - discuss the ways in which smoking affects health;
   - describe two of the major health promotion models used to educate people to stop smoking.
3. *Questions for the student to answer*:
   What are the major ways in which smoking affects health?
   (a) physical

   (b) social

   (c) psychological

   (d) economic

   What are the two major models used in health promotion?

   (i)

   (ii)
4. Further reading

Delivering a lecture

Beitz (1994) has identified six basic steps that are useful to follow before delivering a lecture:

- planning
- writing a detailed outline
- rehearsing
- selecting examples
- knowing the content
- choosing visual aids (see p. 150).

The planning phase.   This incorporates many of the aspects discussed in 'The what of teaching', above. As Beitz (1994) writes, 'A good oral presentation is an inspiring experience in which learners' minds are broadened and their interests piqued'. You may wish to add at this juncture 'and the teacher survives'! It is, however, safe to say that there is a substantial amount of literature available supporting the view that the teacher can learn very useful techniques without too much difficulty (Cooper, 1989).

ACTIVITY 6.15

Imagine that you have been asked to undertake a 1-hour lecture at your local college of nursing. Make a list of all the aspects you think you should include in planning your teaching session. Check your answer against the list already given on page 133.

As identified in Chapter 5, varying your teaching methods will appeal to the students' different learning styles, and even within the lecture, you should try to introduce some change of activity, for example, the use of audiovisual aids or gapped handouts, and allow time for questions during and after the session.

Writing a detailed outline. There is a fine balance to be drawn here. First, it is tempting to write down all that you know on a particular subject and then read it to the group. This should be avoided at all costs as it does not allow for student interaction and potentially makes the teaching session both short and boring. Furthermore, it gives the impression that the teacher wants to control the learners rather than learning alongside them.

The preparation of teaching notes will help you to start planning your teaching session. You will find that the preparation is initially extremely time-consuming but becomes much quicker with practice. The plans can also be updated. This means that they can be used again, and, as a result, your material is gradually built up. They are also a very useful prompt in the teaching situation and will keep your teaching on course.

1. Keep your notes reasonably short, but always include the outcomes or objectives for the session and explain their relevance.
2. Highlight important points on your plan by using a highlighter pen or red ink. This will ensure you do not omit any information that is crucial to your teaching.
3. Fasten your papers together securely or ensure that they are adequately numbered. (If you are extremely nervous and drop them, you will want to be able to reorder them quickly!)
4. Make sure that your plan follows a logical sequence, with a clear introduction, middle and end. Use the introduction to outline what you intend to do and its relevance, the middle section to provide the new information, and the summary to 'pull together' the main points.

Rehearsing. There are unfortunately no short cuts to this aspect as timing is crucial if teaching is to be effective. Many of us have, unfortunately, experienced the teaching session that has run way over time, leaving the students tense, irritable and totally switched off. The answer to this potential problem lies in rehearsal, possibly in front of a friend with a willing ear. The confidence that you can gain from doing this is tremendous. First, it enables you to become much more conversant with your subject matter, and second, it ensures that you will not run out of material in the first 5 minutes.

Selecting examples. This involves choosing practical examples from your own area of work. For example, if a community nurse is teaching on the subject of the safe storage of drugs in the client's home, it becomes much more meaningful to the student if this can be applied to her own experiences. This helps to bring 'teaching to life'.

When planning your presentation, it is always worth asking yourself what relevant examples you can use to link theory with practice. To add a note of caution in selecting examples, beware of relying too heavily on stories from your own practice unless they are totally pertinent to what you are teaching.

Knowing the content. This is probably the only aspect in which no amount of strategic planning will help; you must have an understanding of your subject material and the major concepts involved. Beitz (1994) argues that a willingness to share with the students the learning strategies you have used to assimilate the material may aid their understanding.

It is also useful (and will save you from embarrassment) if you have a reserve of knowledge over and above that which you are going to teach. By doing this, you will not be worried by most questions the group may raise. On the other hand, there is no disgrace in a teacher not knowing the answer to a question, and to say so is far preferable to 'bluffing' your way through. Thankfully, the days when a teacher was expected to know everything are long gone.

Discussion and tutorial groups

These groups are best used when there are small groups of students. Between 12 and 15 students is ideal as larger numbers make it difficult for individual contributions. All of the methods are useful in enabling students to develop their skills in decision-making.

Tutorial groups

These are usually used as a 'back-up' to information already being given by other methods. For example, a tutorial group may look at specific issues that have been raised during a lecture or want to discuss the best way in which they can prepare themselves for an important examination. These groups are teacher led, and the teacher needs a good understanding of what is to be discussed to enable the students to reach their conclusions.

Small group discussions

Small group discussions are best suited to the following activities:

- brainstorming
- snowballing
- buzz groups
- the presentation of projects or assignments
- problem-solving.

Brainstorming.   This is a way of collecting ideas from all of the individuals in the group on how to deal with a particular problem. The students literally shout out their ideas on a particular issue, and these are then written down without comment or discussion.

Abbatt and McMahon (1993) identify four distinct phases of the brainstorming exercise. If learning is to take place, the teacher must be clear as to the problem or the ideas that she is trying to produce.

- *Phase 1*. This involves the need for all of the group to be clear on the types of idea that they are being asked to produce. Examples might be:

  - What are the advantages and disadvantages of using the lecture as a teaching method?
  - What factors might encourage a patient to stop smoking?

- *Phase 2*. The facilitator of the group (teacher or student) asks the group for suggestions and then writes them on the board as quickly as possible. No idea is excluded from the exercise, regardless of how irrelevant it may appear. By the same token, ideas should be recorded even if they have been previously suggested. No comment or discussion is entered into at this stage.

■ *Phase 3*. All of the suggestions are examined to ensure that there is a common understanding within the group of all the issues raised, and also to dispense with any of the ideas that the group feel to be inappropriate or do not wish to discuss.

■ *Phase 4*. All of the remaining ideas are then discussed fully and used to resolve the problem.

Brainstorming is a very useful method of enabling individual students to increase in confidence within the group. The speed at which the activity is undertaken does not allow the student to consider how her idea will be received by the rest of the group and also enables students further to develop someone else's idea.

Snowballing.   This method involves the initial discussion of a subject in small groups, which then develops into a discussion in larger groups (just like a snowball that increases in size as it is rolled). This method has the added advantage that it can be used in larger groups of up to 32 students as long as space is available.

The process starts with a clear statement of what is wanted from the group, for example, how can we help to ensure patients' and their visitors' personal safety while they are in hospital? Time is then given for each student to think about the issues individually. Their ideas are then combined with those of another student, and between them, they identify the similarities and differences in their ideas and what, if anything, they wish to reject. The pairs then 'snowball' into groups of 4, 8 and then 16, during which the issues are compared and discussed until a comprehensive answer is reached.

This is a particularly useful exercise if you are teaching a controversial subject, for example the banning of smoking in all public places, as one group may have to persuade another that their ideas are the 'right' ones.

Buzz groups.   Students are divided into small groups of between 2 and 6, and each is asked to discuss issues for a short period of time. An appointed reporter (often called a rapporteur) then feeds the information back to the group as a whole. To use the effects of smoking on health as an example, one group could be asked what the physical effects would be, one group the social effects, and so on.

Project presentations.   This is a useful method for you to employ if the subject you are teaching involves the discovery of information. For example, it may be about the function of a voluntary organisation that has been set up to support patients, or about drawing up a community profile. Students can work either singly or in groups and the information gained is presented and shared with the whole of the group, usually using audiovisual equipment.

The methods discussed so far are extremely useful in helping the quieter members of the group to grow in confidence and in helping them to develop their interpersonal skills.

All of the above have two crucial elements that you, as the teacher, need to consider. First, the purpose of the session should be clear to the students, and second, the students should feel comfortable and safe enough to contribute; for example, they should not feel that they are going to be made to look foolish in front of the group. There is undoubtedly an art in facilitating discussion groups that enables the teacher to support and get the best out of the students; this comes largely with experience.

Seminars

This method is particularly student centred as it involves the student presenting either a paper or an essay, following which a group discussion takes place. It is a very useful method for exploring issues of a sociological nature, for example, the effects of social class on health, or ethical decision-making. While you as a teacher, need a sound understanding of the subject material, it is useful to ask the student to formulate two or three questions from the paper, which can then be discussed by the group.

ACTIVITY 6.16

What aspects of teaching from your particular area of practice do you think would be best taught using the group discussion methods?

Role play

Role play is extremely useful in developing problem-solving skills and communication strategies, and in trying to change students' attitudes. It involves students playing the part of other people in a situation previously identified by the teacher. Jarvis (1988) has identified that role play encourages active participation, enables problems of human behaviour and relationships to be presented and helps students to understand the relationship between the way in which they think and feel. It is believed that, because the students have a clearer understanding of themselves, it makes them more aware of the 'roles' adopted by the patients and clients in their care.

However, the use of role play as a teaching method has been criticised as being unreal (Munroe et al, 1983). The problems enacted may be artificial representations of real events, and students may exaggerate the roles so that they bear little resemblance to reality.

ACTIVITY 6.17

Think about your own learning experience. Have you taken part in a role play exercise? If so, did you find the experience enjoyable? If not, why do you think this was?

You will probably have identified that you found the experience extremely stressful for many reasons, First, the fact that you are required to 'act' in front of the group is particularly daunting. Second, you are required to 'make it up as you go along', and third, you may have been asked to enact a role that you had difficulty in relating to. I was once asked to take on the role of a Minister of War. As someone totally opposed to violence, I had extreme problems! It is, therefore, of vital importance when planning a role play exercise, that the students' are comfortable with the process and you, as a teacher, are sensitive to their needs.

There are some key steps you may wish to take when planning your role play.

- Identify clearly what you want the students to learn from the exercise.
- Provide the students with clear guidelines on the character they are to play and his or her background.
- Keep the situation relatively simple, with no more than four players. The teacher can miss some very important issues when she comes to summarise if it is too complex.
- Give the role players time for preparation.
- Explain clearly to the audience the purpose of the session.
- Discuss fully with the group the key issues raised in the role play.

Box 6.5 Contains an example of role play and how it may assist learning. This scenario could be used to teach the students the communication skills required when faced with behaviour that is difficult to deal with in practice.

BOX 6.5	*An example of role play*

A lady telephones the ward and demands to know why her admission has been cancelled. She is extremely angry.

The information given to student A would be as follows: You are a 55-year-old lady who has been on the waiting list for 9 months to have your gallbladder removed. You are frequently in a great deal of pain. You have just opened your morning's post to discover that the operation you were due to have the day after tomorrow has been cancelled for the second time. This is despite the fact that you contacted the ward yesterday to confirm that it would go ahead and, as a result, have reorganised your work commitments.

The information given to student B would be: You are in charge on a very busy surgical ward. The student nurse comes to tell you that there is a lady on the phone who is very angry. The student tells you that it seems that the lady was expecting to be admitted to the ward tomorrow for an operation and wants to know what's going on.

Learning from critical incidents

These are often used in the classroom situation in order to develop reflective practice. Smith and Russell (1991, p. 287) provide an excellent example of the application of reflective practice to the teaching situation that involved the use of a journal:

> Everyone was very busy. Sister told me to take his wife a cup of tea and sit with her: the doctor would see her shortly. She didn't know her husband had died. I felt sick. Mrs X asked me how her husband was. I kept saying I didn't know what had happened but that the doctor would come soon and let her know. I was frightened she would know I was lying. I wished the doctor would hurry.

This experience was then used in the classroom to discuss issues relating to communication, care of both people who are dying and their relatives and stress in nursing.

Independent/directed learning

Based on your own experience, you will have your own views about self-directed or independent learning. There are a variety of views on its appropriateness as a teaching method.

It is likely that, in the past, you have been taught using the self-directed/independent method. How useful did you find this in terms of your own learning? If you did not find that the method helped you to learn, why was this?

There are two key elements to self-directed/independent learning that must be acknowledged if learning is to be effective:

1. The students take increasing responsibility for achieving the learning objectives or outcomes.
2. Students work at their own pace.

Fundamental to self-directed study is the need for adequate facilities, for example, library and information technology, since most criticisms directed at this approach to learning are centred around the lack of resources. This is not always the case, however, and entire programmes of study are increasingly being developed using this method. The level of student independence is largely determined by the course planners who identify what is to be learned and how it is to be learned.

In view of this, there are degrees of self-directed/independent learning. Ewan and White (1996, p. 97) provide a very useful table that identifies the stages occurring in the transition from learning being totally teacher directed to being totally student directed. It is recognised that courses leading to a nationally recognised qualification are rarely totally self-directed. This is particularly so in preregistration courses in nursing.

Why do you think this may be so?

The main reason that preregistration courses in nursing are not totally student directed is largely because of the criteria set down by the **statutory bodies** in nursing in order to maintain standards and patient safety.

Think about your current role. Make a list of the activities that you think could be taught wholly self-directed, partly self-directed or teacher directed.

Self-directed learners become more experienced in working without close supervision so that when they enter their jobs as nurses they are more confident of their own abilities and do not have to rely on someone else to tell them what to do. (Ewan and White, 1996, p. 98)

ACTIVITY 6.21

Looking back on your previous experience, do you think that Ewan and White are correct in holding this view. If so, why?

Ewan and White go on to say that you, as the teacher, must try to help students recognise the importance of what they can contribute to their own and other students' learning.

ACTIVITY 6.22

How do you think you can achieve this in your own teaching?

You may have identified some of the following points:

■ the need to know your students well
■ treating them with respect
■ helping them to identify their own learning needs
■ acknowledging that you value their views
■ trying to ensure adequate resources.

Experiential learning

As a practitioner involved in teaching, it is likely that much of the learning that takes place in the students for whom you have responsibility occurs experientially.

ACTIVITY 6.23

What do you understand by the term 'experiential learning'?

Experiential learning, according to Burnard (1990), contains five key elements:

1. There is an emphasis on personal experience.
2. It is an active process.
3. Students are encouraged to reflect, and therefore, learn from their own experiences.
4. Experience is valued as a learning episode in itself.
5. The facilitator/teacher adopts a supportive role in the learning process.

It is clear from the above that the area of practice is the prime place for this type of learning to occur.

Consider how you as a practitioner can facilitate the experiential learning of the students whom you have been allocated. What factors do you think are important?

You have probably identified aspects such as your own current knowledge and experience, the time available within your current role to support the student, and your knowledge of what the student already knows in terms of theory. It is important at this stage to note that while curricula in nurse education combine theory and practice, the theory does not always come before the practice, and students can learn equally well by gaining some of their experience in practice and then learning the theory that underpins it. For example, it is possible for a student to be able to undertake a blood pressure recording safely without having a full understanding of the theory relating to hypertension.

Audiovisual aids

There are many types of aid to help you in your teaching. First, it is useful to identify their value and purpose. Audiovisual aids and technology have several functions. They:

- enhance clarity of communication
- provide diversity in teaching methods
- aid retention
- give impact
- provide experience not normally available
- simulate real-life situations
- permit practice and thus give confidence
- use a range of senses
- increase and sustain attention
- provide realism
- increase the meaningfulness of abstract concepts.

Most colleges of nursing have their own department that will be able to offer specific advice. While the following list is not exhaustive, it will provide you with an overview of what is available:

- chalkboards – it is worth remembering that these are not easy to write on if you have never practised
- white boards
- felt and magnetic boards
- Interactive videos/computerised programmes
- charts and models
- broadcasts
- tape-recordings
- films
- film strips
- slide projectors.

When deciding whether to use an audiovisual aid, remember that it should not be used as an optional extra or as the provider of the whole of the teaching that is to take place.

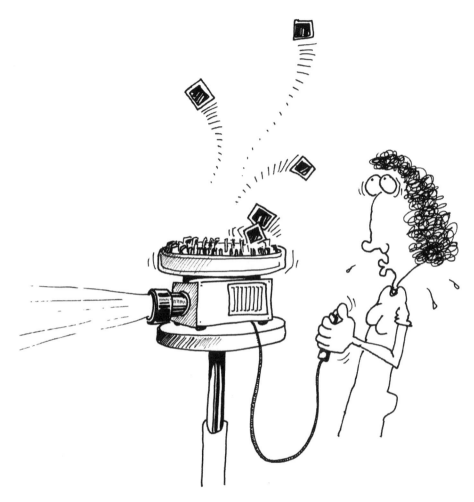

Audiovisual aids

There are some fundamental questions to ask yourself before you make a final decision about the sort of audiovisual aid you want to use. Indeed, there are many other ways of helping students to retain information, for example, field trips which are often an extremely enjoyable way of learning. It is crucial, however, that any visit is relevant to the learning and the theory that underpins it. For example, students early in their studies gain tremendous benefit from discussing the concepts of primary health care in the college setting and then following this up by a guided tour around a local health centre. To refer back to the theory given in Chapter 5, the experience must be *meaningful* for the student if learning is to take place.

If your choice of teaching method is a lesson or lecture, overhead transparencies are a very useful aid to the session. The use of 'acetates' clarifies the key points for students and assists them to make notes. They also have an added advantage for the nervous teacher in that their use diverts the attention from the teacher to the screen. There are some basic rules to follow in preparing your overhead transparencies, which are incorporated into the following 10-point plan:

1. Always use letters at least 1 cm high.
2. Never use ordinary typewritten copy. It is far too small for anyone sitting beyond the front row to see.
3. If you are preparing your overheads by hand, always use a strong base colour. For example, black and blue show up clearly. The colour red is particularly difficult to see on an overhead projector. Note that some projectors enable you to draw diagrams as you speak.
4. Always switch off the projector between use or when you have finished. It is not only a strain on the eyes but also an assault on the ears of students, particularly when using older machinery.
5. Never put too many words on the transparency. Six lines is probably the maximum for it not to look crowded.
6. Resist the temptation to talk to the projector and ignore the students.
7. Reveal information on the overhead one point at a time. This will prevent students from writing everything down before they have had a chance to assimilate the information you are presenting. If you cover part of the acetate with a sheet of paper, note that, standing by the equipment, you will still be able to read the words on the acetate.
8. Never put all of your teaching material on overheads. Not only is it very boring for students, but it will also make your teaching stilted and unspontaneous. Furthermore, the students will be exhausted.
9. Give students time to write notes from the overheads. Remember, a minute of silence is a long time for you but not for the student who is trying to copy what you have written.
10. Provide evidence for what you are saying.

Finally, always have a back-up plan of action. You may need this if the light bulb 'blows' in the projector. In order to save students from having to copy down what is on your transparencies, you may want to prepare handouts of the content. These can, if all goes well, be given out at the end. However, in the event of faulty equipment, you can use the handouts as a framework for your session. Remember, if you do prepare handouts, do tell the students at the start of the class that these are available to save them trying to copy everything down.

TEACHING A SKILL

As a practitioner, teaching skills are probably an important aspect of our role, either in teaching patients/clients to undertake a particular procedure for themselves or teaching student nurses skills, such as the safe moving and handling of patients.

As experienced practitioners, many of the skills that you undertake in your daily work, for example, the positioning of your feet prior to moving a patient, are largely carried out subconsciously. It is likely that, because of the amount of practice you have had at doing the procedure, it has become instinctive.

We have learned from earlier chapters in this book that learning is enhanced if the material is provided in a logical sequence. This is particularly relevant when teaching a skill as the action can be broken down into a series of stages or steps. Skills teaching involves learning in both the cognitive and the motor domains.

Imagine that you have a new student nurse on your ward and you want to teach her the safe administration of drugs from the trolley. Write down the steps you would need to go through in order to complete the task safely.

You will want to check the following items, although their order may change depending on your individual preference:

- the drug bottle label against the patient's drug administration record
- the dosage of the drug
- the time the drug is to be given
- that it is being given to the correct patient by asking him
- the name on the patient's armband to confirm this
- that the patient does not have any allergies to the drug about to be given.

If skills can be broken down as a series of steps, they are much more easily understood by the student, although there are other factors for us to consider, for example, the level of motivation of the student and how the subject is presented by the teacher.

EVALUATING THE EFFECTIVENESS OF YOUR TEACHING

The process of evaluating teaching and learning is addressed separately in this book, in chapter 7, particularly in relation to assessment and student feedback. This section will look specifically at the different evaluation methods you may wish to adopt before, during and after delivering your teaching session.

Purpose

When evaluating a teaching session, many of the headings identified previously in preparing your lesson plan can be utilised. For example, what exactly are you going to evaluate and, probably more importantly, why? This is crucial as it will ultimately determine the strategy that you adopt. At this point you may wish to skim through Chapter 7.

Make a list of the benefits that you feel can be gained for both learners and teachers by evaluating your teaching.

Under the 'student' heading you may have included aspects such as the 'feel-good factor'. The fact that the teacher is openly evaluating the effectiveness of her teaching often acts as a motivator, also providing the student with a clear picture of what she has learned.

For the teacher, evaluation provides an excellent framework for improving the session. For example, you may have incorporated role play into your session and, following evaluation, now feel that a discussion group would have been more appropriate in order to meet your objectives.

Kiger (1995, p. 221) states that 'evaluation is an inevitable and essential part of the teaching – learning process.'

ACTIVITY 6.27

What do you think Kiger meant by the above statement? What does the statement mean to you? You may find it helpful to consider why it is both inevitable and essential.

You may have included issues such as the students' opinion of the value of the teaching session or whether the teacher felt that she had explained the subject in a way that was easily understood. Kiger terms this 'informal evaluation' and suggests that this takes place regardless of any strategic plan.

Abbatt and McMahon (1993) identify three aspects that can be effectively evaluated by the teacher: the plan, the process and the product.

Evaluating the teaching plan

This involves all of the preparation undertaken by the teacher prior to the teaching taking place. This may be a 'one-off' teaching session, in either the practice or college environment, or a full course or module. It may appear almost contradictory to talk about evaluating a teaching session before it has begun, but there are many aspects of teaching that will greatly increase the likelihood of the content of the session or course being appropriate. To this end, there are some fundamental questions that you can ask once you have amassed your teaching material and clearly written your plan.

- Have you considered and included any instructions you have been given? For example, the session may be one of a sequence. If so, does your preparation follow on logically from the foregoing session and lead logically on to the next?
- Can you fulfil the objectives you have set for yourself with the content of the session?
- Will you be able to complete the teaching session in the time that you have been allocated?
- Is your teaching pitched at the right level for the group or student you are about to teach? For example, you would expect a student nurse in the third year of the course to have a greater understanding of how to care for an unconscious patient than a student in her first year.

- How confident are you with the teaching methods you will use? From previous chapters, it is clear that using a variety of teaching methods both enhances the learning process and leads to a much more enjoyable learning experience.
- Are your objectives sufficiently clear to ensure that the student understands what is to be gained from the session?

ACTIVITY 6.28

Refer back to the work you undertook in Activity 6.12. Think how you could find out if you have fulfilled your objectives.

The most straightforward answer to this is probably to ask the students. For example, you can pose a question directly relating to the objective and hope for an appropriate response. It is crucial to acknowledge, however, that it may only tell you that one student, or however many answer the question correctly, has an understanding, but does not tell you about the whole class. Generally speaking, it is extremely valuable to use the first 5–10 minutes of any teaching session discussing with the students what they can expect to gain from it.

Evaluating the teaching process

Abbatt and McMahon (1993) argue that evaluation of the process of teaching centres largely around observation and discussion. Before these aspects are developed in relation to your teaching plan, however, it may be useful to identify what is actually meant by the process of teaching. A straightforward definition of process (*Concise Oxford Dictionary*, 1983) is the 'state of going on or being carried on'. From this, you might conclude that this type of evaluation can take place during the time the subject material is being delivered.

A great deal of information can be gained in evaluating the process of teaching by the use of observation. This may be by the teacher delivering the teaching session or by other teachers, when it is known as **peer review**.

Use of checklists/questionnaires in evaluation

A checklist is an extremely useful guide in enabling you to identify aspects of your teaching that you could improve, and it is particularly fruitful when used at the same time as students' written evaluations.

ACTIVITY 6.29

Imagine that you have just delivered a teaching session on your specialist subject area. Identify some questions that you would want to ask about the effectiveness of your teaching.

There are many evaluation tools available to assist you in this, all of which identify five or six key areas for evaluation (Box 6.6).

BOX 6.6	*Areas for evaluation*

1. The teacher's presentation of the subject material. This involves the practical aspects of subject delivery, for example:
   - Could the teacher be heard?
   - Did the teaching follow a logical progression?
   - Was it delivered in words that the students understood?
   - Were the visual aids used clear and appropriate?

2. The teacher's approach to the students. This includes questions such as:
   - Was the teacher enthusiastic about the subject?
   - Was the teacher able to establish a rapport with the students?
   - Was the teacher able to recognise the need for student participation?
   - Did the teacher respond sensitively to the students?

3. Student understanding and participation.
   - Were the students encouraged to become actively involved in the teaching session?
   - Was the learning related to the students' previous experience?
   - Was student interest maintained?
   - Was the students' level of knowledge elicited at the start in order to build on this?

4. Meeting objectives:
   - Were the objectives for the session discussed with the students?
   - Was the choice of objectives appropriate?
   - Were the objectives specific and unambiguous?
   - Were the objectives shared with the students?

5. The teaching and learning environment:
   - Was the general environment conducive to learning, for example, not too hot, too cold or too small?
   - Were surrounding noise levels acceptable?
   - Were the furnishings and teaching aids of an acceptable standard?

6. Feedback:
   - Were students given immediate, appropriate and unambiguous feedback on the points they raised during the session?
   - Were students advised on how they could improve or find out more information?

Using the list in Box 6.6 as a framework, you should be able to develop your own evaluation tool, which can then be adapted to meet any teaching situation, either in the classroom or practice setting, and with individuals or groups.

Evaluating the teaching product

This type of evaluation tends to be more relevant to a course or module as it involves more formal assessment and examination processes. For example, a high pass rate at examination is a reasonably good indicator that the product is satisfactory and that the criteria laid down for it are being met. Whatever the type of evaluation used, there is one aspect that is fundamental to them all, that is, the need to act on the findings in order to improve the way in which we teach.

While the above short section should provide a practical aid in helping you to evaluate your teaching, a much fuller picture is provided in Chapter 7.

CONCLUSION

This chapter has provided you with the basic information that you will need in order for you to teach effectively, either in your area of practice or in the classroom. It is not intended that the chapter provides you with an in-depth knowledge of the process of teaching and learning, but it should act as a reference point to get you started. The use of learning outcomes or objectives provides you with a useful framework on which to build your teaching, particularly if you are new to the role. We hope that it will be a useful resource.

GLOSSARY

Action learning: a form of learning by experiencing and solving real problems, usually as they occur, for example, in the work place.

Curriculum design: the grouping of topics or subjects in a way in which they can be easily understood, for example, as anatomy and physiology, and health promotion.

Curriculum model: a framework for the ways in which individuals learn (see Chapter 1).

Facilitator: one who enables students to learn by supporting and guiding as opposed to teaching formally.

Mentor: an adviser; the term is sometimes used interchangeably with that of supervisor.

Peer review: a way of evaluating your performance using colleagues of similar status to carry out the review.

Philosophy: the underpinning beliefs and values of a system or process.

Statutory body: in nursing, this relates to the four National Boards responsible for validating nursing programmes in the four countries of the UK.

REFERENCES

Abbatt F and McMahon R (1993) *Teaching Healthcare Workers: A Practical Guide*, 2nd edn. London: Macmillan.

Alexander MF (1982) Integrating theory and practice in nursing – 1. *Nursing Times*, 78(17), 65–68.

Baldwin A (1977) *One-to-One*. New York: Evans & Co.

Beitz M (1994) Dynamics of effective oral presentations: strategies for nurse educators. *AORN Journal*, **59**(5), 1026–1032.

Boud D, Keogh R and Walker D (1985) *Reflections: Training Experience into Learning*. London: Kogan Page.

Burnard P (1990) *Learning Human Skills: An Experimental Guide for Nurses*, 2nd edn. Oxford: Heinemann.

Burrel T (1988) *Curriculum Design and*

Development. London: Prentice Hall.

Clifford C (1995) The role of the nurse teachers: concerns, conflicts and challenges. *Nurse Education Today*, **15**, 11–16.

Concise Oxford Dictionary (1983) Oxford: Oxford University Press.

Cooper SS (1989) Teaching tips: some lecturing do's and don'ts. *Journal of Continuing Education in Nursing*, **20**, 140–141.

Curzio J (1997) A plan for introducing evidence based practice *Nursing Times*, **93**(52), 55–56.

Curzon LB (1985) *Teaching in Further Education. An Outline of Principles and Practice*, 3rd edn. Eastbourne: Holt Rinehart & Winston.

Dewing J (1990) Reflective practice. *Senior Nurse*, **10**(10), 26–28.

Ewan C and White R (1996) *Teaching Nursing. A Self Instructional Handbook*, 2nd edn. London: Chapman & Hall.

Ghaye T (1996) *An Introduction to Learning Through Critical Reflective Practice*. Newcastle upon Tyne: Pentaxion.

Jarvis P (1988) *Adult and Continuing Education – Theory and Practice*. London: Routledge.

Jolly U (1997) *The First-year Nurse Tutor: A Qualitative Study*. Salisbury, Wiltshire: Mark Allen.

Kiger AM (1995) *Teaching for Health*, 2nd edn. New York: Churchill Livingstone.

Knowles M (1984) *Androgogy in Action*. San Francisco: Jossey Bass.

McCaugherty D (1992) Integrating theory and practice. *Senior Nurse*, **13**(4), 28–29.

Munroe EA, Manthei R and Small JJ (1983) *Counselling Skills Approach*. New Zealand: Methuen.

Parkin C (1989) Humor, health, and higher education: laughing matters. *Journal of Nurse Education*, **28**, 229–230.

Prognoff I (1975) *Journal Workshop*. New York: Dialogue House Library.

Quinn F (1994) *The Principles and Practice of Nurse Education*, 2nd edn. London: Chapman & Hall.

Rogers C (1983) *Freedom to Learn for the 80's*. Columbus' OH: Charles E Merrill.

Shields E (1994) A daily dose of reflection. Developing skills through journal writing. *Professional Nurse*, Aug, 755–759.

Smith A and Russell J (1991) Using critical learning incidents in nurse education. *Nurse Education Today*, **11**, 284–291.

United Kingdom Central Council for Nursing, Midwifery and Health Visiting (1992) *Code of Professional Conduct for Nurses, Midwives and Health Visitors*. London: UKCC.

FURTHER READING

Brown S, Earlam C and Race P (1995) *500 Tips for Teachers*. London: Kogan Page. *This is a superb book to dip into, which will give you confidence prior to commencing your teaching session. It outlines many practical ways of ensuring that your teaching is effective, and it is presented in a very readable format.*

Forsyth I, Jolliffe A and Stevens D (1995) *Preparing a Course*. London: Kogan Page. *This is one of a series of books by the above authors that forms a complete guide to teaching a course. Other titles are: Planning a Course, Delivering a Course and Evaluating a Course. As the titles suggest, they are primarily aimed at teaching at course level, but the content of all four books is extremely relevant to practitioners undertaking teaching, and they are very readable.*

Jarvis P and Gibson S (1997) *The Teacher Practitioner and Mentor in Nursing, Midwifery, Health Visiting and Social Services*, 2nd edn. London: Stanley Thornes. *This book explores the roles of the teacher–practitioner and mentor. It includes many important aspects such as the teacher–learner relationship and interpersonal skills. It also contains a useful section on mentoring.*

Rowntree D (1994) *Preparing Materials for Open, Distance and Flexible Learning*. London: Kogan Page. *The text identifies the sequence required in order to develop materials for open, distance and flexible learners. It is particularly useful as it provides checklists to ensure that your material is both appropriate and effective.*

7 The evaluation of learning and teaching

Anne Eaton

INTRODUCTION

The terms 'assessment' and 'evaluation' are often used interchangeably, yet they are fundamentally different. In Chapter 4, the term 'assessment' was defined for you.

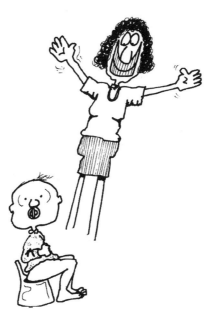

The evaluation of learning and teaching

Define the term 'evaluation'. Now write down how you think this differs from the definition of 'assessment.'

As will be seen later in this chapter, assessment can be defined as the measurement of learning, and evaluation can be defined as measuring the effectiveness of learning and teaching.

Although you are probably undertaking the role of teacher and assessor in clinical practice, you are also a learner in this situation, and the evaluation processes outlined in the chapter will therefore apply to you in both areas, that is, your teaching and your learning. However, as a teacher, you will need to evaluate individually and contribute to the evaluation of the learners in your clinical environment, and you will, therefore, be evaluating *their* learning.

LEARNING OBJECTIVES

After reading this chapter, you should be able to:

- define evaluation
- differentiate between assessment and evaluation
- give examples of different methods of evaluation
- evaluate your own teaching and learning
- evaluate the learning of others in your clinical environment.

Ellington et al (1993) distinguish between the concepts of assessment and evaluation as shown in Box 7.1.

BOX 7.1	*Assessment and evaluation (Ellington et al, 1993)*
	1. Assessment measures student learning, which is achieved as a result of a teaching/learning situation
	2. Evaluation is a series of activities that are designed to measure the effectiveness of a teaching/learning system as a whole

Alternatively, assessment can be defined as the collection of data on which we can base evaluation. As previously identified in Chapter 4, assessment can be seen to be descriptive and objective; that is, if another assessor were to undertake the job of assessing the same item, the findings should be the same.

Evaluation could also be seen as the process of making personalised judgements and decisions about achievements, about expectations and about the effectiveness and value of what we are doing. Evaluation involves ideas about 'good' and 'bad' teaching and learning. That is, it relates to its worth, and these ideas are based upon the evaluator's own ideology.

To extend the discussion on these two areas, it can be suggested that assessment is value-free, objective and, on the whole, **criterion referenced**, that is, assessment of work using a set of standards or criteria. On the other hand, evaluation is a value judgemental concept and involves examining and judging, concerning the quality, significance, amount, degree or condition of something. In your case, that 'something' will be the processes that your learners have gone through and that you have assessed – your teaching and learning, and their learning.

Thus we can see that the assessment of learners forms the major part of the evaluation process, and the outcomes of both should identify not only learning achieved by the individual, but also an educational programme, be it delivered in the classroom or the workplace, that fits the purpose. Remember that, as in the nursing process, evaluation is one of four components: assessment, planning, implementation and evaluation. You can apply these components to your role as teacher and assessor.

This does not mean that evaluation occurs only at the end of a learning experience but rather, that evaluation is ongoing and vital to the development and evolution of learning and teaching. The ultimate outcome of evaluation is decision-making, that is, identifying what needs to be changed and changing it. This then leads back into the cycle of activity and on to the assessment of learning needs. The intention of evaluation is to make conscious what most of us do much of the time as part of the process of teaching (Rogers, 1994).

Evaluation may be one of the more difficult skills required of you in your role as teacher, and it is important that the techniques involved in evaluation, and indeed the whole process, are developed consciously.

Within your clinical area, and with the many learners whom you come across in your work activities, there is no point in evaluating your teaching, and the learning that has taken place, if you are not prepared to change what you do as a result of the feedback that the evaluation process gives you. Evaluation can only be effective if you are prepared to stop the existing programme when a problem is detected and redevelop your teaching accordingly. However, it would be foolhardy and impulsive to act immediately on the results of one evaluation that may identify a relatively minor problem. It is more appropriate to wait and see whether subsequent evaluations give the same results; if so, *then* is the time to change the offending part of the programme. If action is taken too early, change may be made when change is not necessary. With each successive cycle of evaluation, the processes of teaching and learning should become progressively more refined, and the ultimate results should become more effective and efficient.

ACTIVITY 7.2

Can you think of an aspect of your teaching that you:
■ changed when it was not necessary
■ did not change when it did prove necessary?

In my own experience, I changed my teaching of recording blood pressure when one learner could not grasp the skill, only eventually to identify that the failure to learn lay, in fact, with the learner. Conversely, I maintained another session because I felt comfortable with it when it was obvious from learner assessment that very few of the group were learning.

To develop the notion of evaluating learning and teaching, we need to explore the questions:

- Why evaluate?
- When to evaluate?
- Where to evaluate?
- What to evaluate?
- Who to evaluate?
- How to evaluate?

WHY EVALUATE?

We all need to evaluate many aspects of our personal as well as our working lives. You might evaluate how well your coat was cleaned by the dry cleaners or how effective you think your son's new teacher is; or you may evaluate the delivery of client care or the process of teaching and learning. In the latter areas, the purpose of any evaluation process is to improve upon outcomes, teaching processes or learning achievement and ultimately to benefit patient/client care. In our present health service, however, we may also need to evaluate to ensure the cost-effectiveness of the delivery of learning. In some circumstances, an evaluation process that identifies poor learning or poor client care may mean that drastic measures need to be taken, such as stopping an education programme or withdrawing learners from a particular care environment. We may also need to submit a formal evaluation of teaching and learning in order to fulfil the requirements of specific educational programmes.

The process of evaluating teaching and learning should show up whether or not the teaching methods used were appropriate, whether the strategy to deliver the programme fitted the situation, whether the assessment methods used were the best choice for the topic or outcomes being assessed and, indeed, whether the learning outcomes had been developed correctly.

Evaluation may illustrate different aspects of what has been taught and what has been learned. It may demonstrate that the two do not match, and, as has been suggested in Chapter 4, failure to learn may result from a failure in the teaching process rather than a failure in the learning process. The process of evaluation provides everyone concerned with the information necessary to move forward.

Nothing is constant; all things evolve – frequently after being evaluated in some way or another.

WHEN TO EVALUATE?

Evaluation is sometimes seen as the end of a process. In reality, it is part of a circular process to which there is no end, but where the results of evaluation lead back to the assessment, or reassessment of a situation, for example, patients'/clients' care needs or a learner's needs within an educational programme (Fig. 7.1).

However, it could be argued that when and how frequently to evaluate depends upon what and how much is being taught and learned, and, in practical terms, on the time available to teach and learn. For example, a nursing student may only be with you for a very short period of time, but his learning, while on placement, needs not only to be assessed, but also evaluated. This could lead to

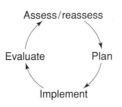

Fig 7.1 *The evaluation cycle.*

repeated, rather superficial evaluation. On the other hand, if a learner's placement with you is for longer, or if the evaluation is for a permanent member of staff, the process might take much longer and be more individualised. The probable answer, then, to 'when' to evaluate is whenever necessary.

WHERE TO EVALUATE?

The evaluation of teaching and learning should take place wherever teaching and learning occur. Depending on your role, this might be in the clinical setting so you need to tailor your evaluation processes so to reflect this. Remember that evaluation will also be undertaken by all the other people involved with the whole programme of learning, and your evaluation should contribute to the total picture – it is one piece in a jigsaw.

WHAT TO EVALUATE?

There are two facets that need to be addressed in evaluation processes. The first covers the concrete, factual, physical components that can be identified in any teaching and/or learning situation and that are easily measurable. They can be linked to the learning outcomes or criteria pertinent to a programme. As identified in Chapter 4, these are probably best described as the knowledge and skills necessary to perform competently in clinical practice.

ACTIVITY 7.3

Stop for a moment and think about your own area of practice.
Identify three such skills or knowledge components.

In relation to knowledge and skills, there may be tight controls on what is evaluated; for example, within the Scottish or National Vocational Qualification (S/NVQ) awards, the amount, complexity and level of skill and knowledge the learner must achieve before he can be said to be competent are clearly identified. Similar processes are seen in most programmes, and the standards that must be achieved and maintained are often specified; thus, it is easy to measure the extent to which these have been met. This evaluation approach measures output against input and is sometimes termed a **scientific evaluation** (Ellington et al, 1993).

ACTIVITY 7.4

Using your examples identified in Activity 7.3, make a list of inputs (from you) and outputs (from your learners).

The inputs you have listed may include:

■ demonstrations
■ teaching
■ acting as a role model

and the outputs:

■ practice
■ the transferability of skills
■ the transferablity of knowledge.

The other area of evaluation relates to the systems and processes that support and contribute to the fixed components of the programme, in other words, the variables contained within any learning process. This is sometimes called **illuminative evaluation** (Ellington et al, 1993).

ACTIVITY 7.5

List the variables that may fall within this category of evaluation. Don't worry about evaluating them in terms of importance – just jot down what comes into your head.

Your list may start with the learners themselves. As we stressed in Chapter 4, all learners are individuals, with their own needs and idiosyncrasies, and all learners, just like your patients/clients, deserve holistic care in relation to their teaching and learning.

The **learning environment** may also be included in your list, and as you are probably most closely involved with the clinical area, you will be very aware of how the climate can change, sometimes at a moment's notice, often dramatically, and how these changes can affect the results of an evaluation process carried out by learners.

Just think for a moment about how the atmosphere changes when a senior staff member is in a bad mood or a clinical crisis such as a cardiac arrest occurs.

ACTIVITY 7.6

Think of two learners who spent the same length of time with you in your clinical area, but who gave different evaluations of their experiences. Why do you think their evaluations differed?

You may have listed your relationships with individual learners, or the progress made with them, and how this may have affected your 'input' and, therefore, their 'output'. Although it would be ideal to suggest that all learners receive the same 'input' from you, it is unrealistic to expect this, because you, the learner and the environment, are not the same from day to day. An evaluation occurs at a particular moment in time and thus gives us a snapshot of what happened at that time.

As with most learning processes, there may be additional benefits felt and gained by some learners, spin-offs such as increased confidence in their own ability and the improvement of their communication skills. These are all bonuses to achieving the aim of any learning programme, which is to learn what is being taught. The attitudes of learners, including their perceptions and opinions, may also be evaluated within this context, as may the attitudes of other staff involved with the support and teaching of learners. Most evaluation systems will incorporate a mixture of the scientific and illuminative components in order to give a broad and deep understanding of the processes involved and the results achieved.

WHO TO EVALUATE?

As this chapter is entitled 'The Evaluation of Learning and Teaching', it may be obvious that who is being evaluated is you, your learners and, to a lesser extent, the other people involved in the learning process. This also suggests that these people are the ones who undertake the process of evaluation, using methods detailed later in the chapter.

HOW TO EVALUATE TEACHING

There are a number of methods of evaluation that can be used to evaluate teaching and learning, and, as you will find out, most methods can be used for both purposes. However, the aim of this section is to explore the evaluation of teaching.

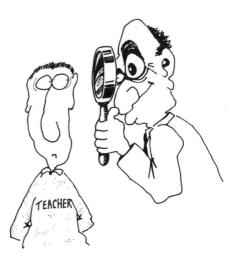

How to evaluate teaching

Self-evaluation

Self-evaluation can help you to identify personal progress, to clarify what is still to be learned and to recognise how past learning can be incorporated into current practices (Burnard, 1988).

If, in your assessment, you identify that some students have failed to learn, then something has gone wrong. It may be that the objectives, learning outcomes or components of the learning contract were unrealistic and did not fit the overall programme aims; or it may be that the methods used to deliver those learning outcomes were inappropriate to the learning style of the individual learner.

Whatever has gone wrong, you need to evaluate your methods and processes in order to identify the problem and correct it in the future. If you do not evaluate yourself, there is a tendency to carry on as usual. The process of self-evaluation allows you to reflect and prepare yourself for future learning.

Within your professional role, you may have a great deal of personal autonomy, together with personal and professional accountability. The autonomy allows you, as an individual, to determine how you practice, within parameters set by, for example, your employer, your linked educational institution and the United Kingdom Central Council for Nursing, Midwifery and Health Visiting (UKCC). This autonomy is a privilege and enables you to develop as an independent practitioner, teacher and assessor within your clinical environment so you need to be rigorous and active in maintaining and developing your standards in these areas (Reece and Walker, 1997). Because of this autonomy, you will be expected to monitor your own standards, and to review and evaluate your own delivery, whether this relates to patient/client care or teaching and assessing learners. This evaluation will enable you to undertake a SWOT or SNOB analysis (Box 7.2).

BOX 7.2	*SWOT or SNOB analysis*

- identify your **S**trengths
- identify your **W**eakness (or **N**eeds)
- Look at the **O**pportunities available
- Consider the **T**hreats (or **B**arriers) that may hinder your delivery or the improvement of your strategies.

ACTIVITY 7.7	

Do a SWOT or SNOB analysis in relation to your role as a teacher.

The thoughts that you might list here will be very personal to you but might include:

- strengths: confidence, enthusiasm, experience
- weaknesses/needs: time, other commitments
- opportunities: working environment, teaching course
- threats/barriers: work demands, other staff.

You are accountable to your learners to offer them the best learning opportunities available for them to learn and progress accordingly.

One way to evaluate yourself is through a self-evaluation (or reflective) diary (see Chapter 6) and through the development of a personal professional portfolio. According to Andrews (1996), reflecting-on-action has two properties in common with evaluation; that is, both are purposeful and active processes. You are involved with updating and expanding your professional development in response to the UKCC's post-registration education and practice (PREP) requirements. It would seem logical to use your development as a teacher and assessor within your clinical environment to fulfil some of these requirements, and a reflective diary, which not only details the processes you have gone through, but also shows how you have learned from these situations and improved your skills, will go some way towards meeting the UKCC's requirements.

Within the publication *PREP and You* (United Kingdom Central Council for Nursing, Midwifery and Health Visiting, 1997), it is suggested that you may wish to work through the following stages when planning your professional portfolio:

1. Review your competence. What are your strengths, areas that you need to develop and areas for further personal development?
2. Set your learning objectives. What do you want to achieve?
3. Develop an action plan. What learning activities will help you to meet your needs?
4. Implement the action plan. Discuss your plan with your manager, link tutor or other relevant personnel.
5. Evaluate what happened. Once you have implemented the action plan, you can think about what happened and what you have learned.
6. Record your study time and learning outcomes. Accurately record all your learning activities.

All of these areas can be addressed in such a way as to encompass your teaching and assessing roles, and the format should enable you to evaluate your techniques, your individual style and your developments in relation to these skills while, at the same time, meeting your PREP requirements.

ACTIVITY 7.8

Using the stages suggested, reflect upon a specific teaching session you have recently given, or plan a session and work through the stages accordingly. Remember that you are specifically looking at your role as a teacher.

Maintaining a personal professional portfolio enables you to keep a record of your professional development, whether in clinical practice, teaching or assessing. However, it is more than a record of achievement, and it should be based upon a regular process of reflection and, by implication, a regular process of evaluation. The benefits of this process are numerous and include the development of analytical skills that you will be able to apply, not only to your own personal and professional growth, but also to the growth of others. Furthermore, such skills help you to assess your current standards of practice and to demonstrate experiential learning, all of which may allow you to obtain credit towards further qualifications.

Within such programmes as the ENB 997/998 and the Training and Development Lead Body NVQ assessor awards, D32 and D33 (see Chapter 4), this process of reflection can help you to evaluate yourself. As well as self-evaluation, others will assess you and go on to evaluate your learning as you will also be observed by the tutors involved with course delivery, and their observation of your session will be documented.

ACTIVITY 7.9

Devise a self-feedback form that you might find useful for *your* assessor to complete in relation to your teaching skills.

Your form may include areas that you feel you need feedback on, such as:

- content
- methods
- timing
- presentation.

Different educational establishments and different programmes mean that varying formats are used to document **trainee teachers'** and **trainee assessors'** progress. Some suggestions are given within the section on evaluation in Chapter 6, but an example of what may be contained within such documentation is given in Box 7.3.

BOX 7.3 | *Example of a practical teaching assessment*

Name: *Joanne French*
Date: *27th August 1998*   Time: *2.30 p.m.*
Clinical area: *Acute male medical ward*
Name of assessor: *Sara Holloway*
Programme undertaken: *ENB 998*
Class/group/individual learner details (e.g. size of group, unit of learning/module, etc.):
Four in group, all nursing students in CFP, first experience in medicine.
Subject/topic:
Drug administration, checking the prescription sheet.
Comments:
Learning objectives set by trainee assessor/teacher:
Clear and well laid out.
Preparation of learners:
All learners were aware of the session and its contents.
Preparation of environment:
Session carried out in the ward seminar room, which had been previously booked. Seating comfortable, though rather formal. Flip chart available, as were blank prescription sheets. Handouts were given to students at the beginning of the session. It may have been more appropriate to give them out at the end.
Relationship with learner(s):
Good relationship, all students relaxed.
Communication skills:

Nervous at first, tended to rush the session and not stick to the lesson plan. Did slow
down eventually.
Knowledge of subject matter:
Very knowledgeable, able to answer students' questions simply.
Application of learning theories:
Aware of theories, beginning to apply to group.
Questioning techniques:
Good technique. Used simple open and closed questions. One question was rather long
and lost the students and the teacher! Did tend to keep asking the same learner.
Feedback:
Gave good positive feedback with no criticisms.
Additional comments by assessor:
Overall, a good session. Some improvement needed in questioning techniques and speed
of delivery.
Comments by trainee assessor/teacher:
I'm glad its over with, but I do need to slow down!
Signed: Assessor   Trainee Assessor/Teacher
Sara Holloway   J. French
Date: 27th August 1998   Date: 27/8/98

Within this section you have looked at evaluating your own teaching and
learning, but you need to examine other ways of evaluating your teaching and
methods of assessing the learning of others in your clinical environment. Some
of these methods can, of course, be used to evaluate patient/client care, but
within your role as teacher and assessor, you need to evaluate whether your
nursing students, health care assistants, newly qualified staff and others have
benefited from their experiences and exposure to learning opportunities within
your clinical environment.

Evaluative feedback can be gained from a number of sources and via a wide
range of methods. In many cases, a whole battery of evaluation techniques are
used in order to gain an overall view of the effectiveness of learning and
teaching. Your evaluation processes will probably relate to a self-contained unit
of learning, which will be specific to your clinical environment and the learners
within it.

The outcome of evaluation should, therefore, aim to identify and demonstrate
the appropriateness of:

- teaching methods
- the structure adopted
- the implementation strategy
- assessment methods
- the learning objectives.

The methods that can be used to ascertain these are:

- checklists
- interviews
- questionnaires
- results from learner assessment
- feedback from other staff.

Using the methods listed above is an individual choice, but it is your responsibility to select the methods best suited to your needs in evaluating your learners and yourself. There is no single correct way to undertake evaluation. The methods selected may differ according to whether you are evaluating the scientific component of a programme or session, evaluating the additional benefits through an illuminative approach or attempting to evaluate both components.

Checklists

Checklists can be used by you to start the self-evaluation process. A checklist should be seen as an *aide-memoire* to the whole process of evaluation and could be likened to **formative assessment**, in which information is gathered to feed into the formal **summative assessment** process.

Most people are relatively familiar with a checklist approach. Think, for example, of when you go shopping and make a list, or when you prepare to undertake a clinical procedure and how you mentally (or physically) tick off the points as you go along. For example, when preparing to undertake an aseptic technique, your list might look like this:

- trolley, appropriately prepared
- dressing pack
- cleansing solution
- strapping
- extra swabs/forceps
- wound swab (just in case!).

ACTIVITY 7.10

Make a checklist of things that you need to ensure you have prepared before you start a teaching session.

Your list may include:

- room booked
- learners aware of session, topic, time and place
- teaching aids available
- learning objectives prepared
- audiovisual aids prepared
- overall session prepared
- self prepared!

This information can be gathered by you before you start a session and fed into the whole evaluative process at the end of the event. The next stage is to deliver the teaching session in question. During this session you will be able to ascertain whether or not the session is going well. As suggested in the section on 'Feedback' in Chapter 4, intrinsic feedback can be gained from your activities; that is, you have an immediate idea how you are performing, using such indicators as the learners' attention and the expression on their faces. This immediate feedback is important, as it might enable you to alter your presentation 'on the hoof', if possible, or take this information into account when evaluating the whole session in order to make alterations for next time.

Interviews

A more formal method that you can use to evaluate your teaching is to question the group concerned or to question individuals from the group. Although this information could be useful, you need to ask specific and objective questions that can be answered by the individuals involved. It may be very difficult for learners to answer questions that need a personal response, especially about you, when they know that they will be working with you again and that you will be assessing their practice. It is best, therefore, if learners' evaluations concentrate on the teaching and learning process rather than on the teachers' competence (Ward-Griffin and Brown, 1992). However, a structured interview may enable you to address some items in greater depth than questionnaires permit, and subsequent questions may develop because of responses to the previous question.

This can be difficult to control at times, and it is all too easy to digress. In order to elicit the information required, it is advisable to prepare your questions in advance and set yourself a time limit for the interview. You will obviously need to record the outcomes of the interview; this could be done using an audiotape, with the learners' permission, or by your making notes during the activity. However, it is difficult to make notes when someone is talking – think back to the time you spent in a classroom, trying to make notes, and listen and understand what was being said, all at the same time. Remember that you must be able to interpret the information later, when the learner is not there to explain what he said or why, so make sure your notes are readable and you can understand them. Adequate preparation beforehand will greatly reduce any problems later.

Questionnaires

It may be more appropriate to devise a questionnaire to distribute to the group, and, by using this method, you may be able to cover more aspects. Your questionnaire can be completed anonymously and be handed in for collation and analysis. The content of the questionnaire must obviously apply to the topic and session concerned but can draw on both the scientific approach and the illuminative approach.

Ideally, you should use both **open questions**, which will need a written, and therefore individual, response, and **closed questions**, which will require only a tick. Closed questions are easier to answer and easier to collate. You are, by using questionnaires as an evaluation method, undertaking research into your teaching, and, by using open and closed questions, you are aiming to collect both **qualitative data** and **quantitative data**.

The key to any questionnaire lies in its response rate (that is, the number of people who actually complete it as a percentage of those to whom it was given). A poor response rate will not give you a fair picture so one way of aiming for a good response rate is to keep your questionnaire simple and answerable.

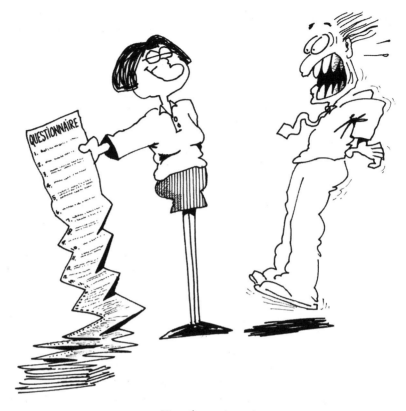

Use of questionnaires

ACTIVITY 7.11

Consider any questionnaires that you have completed in the past. What made some very easy to complete? What made others difficult?

Your responses to the first question might include:

- the length of the questionnaire
- the layout
- the language used

and to the second question, your responses might be:

- too long
- too crowded
- confusing/ambiguous language.

Ideally, a questionnaire should take no longer than 4 or 5 minutes to complete, and telling respondents where to return the questionnaires is vital or you will not get them back. An example of a questionnaire is given in Box 7.4 about a teaching session on recording blood pressures.

BOX 7.4	*Example of a questionnaire*

SESSION: Recording patients' blood pressure
Date: *17th September 1998*
Time: *4.00 p.m.*
Venue: *Seminar room, Ward 1, Gastrointestinal surgery*
Teacher: *Mary Philips*

TOPIC
Please circle one response on the following scales.

(1a) How useful was the taking of each others' blood pressure?
Of little use   1   2   3   4   5   Very useful

(1b) How useful was the demonstration on the patient?
Of little use   1   2   3   4   5   Very useful

(2a) Did you need both demonstrations? (please circle)
    YES   NO

(2b) Please give a reason for the above answer.

(3) Were the demonstrations (please tick one):
Too long?   Too short?   About right?

(4) Were you able to practise the technique?
    YES   NO

(5) Did you feel capable after practice?
    YES   NO

(6) Was the time given to practise:
Too long?   Too short?   Just right?

(7) Were you able to link your skills to what you learned in the classroom about the theory?
    YES   NO

(8) Do you feel confident to undertake the skill on patients/clients?
    YES   NO

DELIVERY
(9) In your opinion, how was the session organised? (please circle)
Poorly   Fairly well   Well   Very well   Excellently

(10) Was the teacher (please circle as appropriate):

Clear	YES	NO
Understandable	YES	NO
Confident	YES	NO
Approachable	YES	NO

(11) Was the environment satisfactory?
    YES   NO

(12) Were handouts and other visual aids satisfactory?
    YES   NO

OVERALL
Please add overleaf any further comments you may feel are useful.

Thank you for your cooperation.

You will need to decide when to distribute your questionnaire, either at the beginning or the end of your session. Whichever way you choose, you need a speedy return of the completed forms, soon after the end of the session, in order to obtain an accurate response from your learners before failing memory or discussion with others can distort or alter the accuracy of their responses.

Once you have collected your completed questionnaires, you will need to collate and analyse the information obtained. You will be collecting both qualitative and quantitative data. Look back at the sample questionnaire (Box 7.4) and identify two questions that will produce quantitative data and two that will lead to qualitative data. Check your responses against the definitions given in the glossary.

In order to analyse accurately and comparatively, it is easier to draw conclusions from information contained within the quantitative data, and you may, therefore, look at ways of transferring your qualitative data into quantitative data.

If you take question 9 in the sample questionnaire (assuming 10 learners in the session), you could transfer the results from the completed question into a blank form as follows:

In your opinion, how was the session organised?

Poorly	Fairly well	Well	Very well	Excellently
		111	11111	11
		(3)	(5)	(2)

You could then surmise that 3 out of 10 respondents, that is, 30%, felt that the session was organised well, and that 5 out of 10, that is, 50% of the learners evaluated that the session had been organised very well. You could then go on to identify the differences in responses and ultimately come to a conclusion about how well, or otherwise, you have organised the session in question.

Once you have collected, collated and analysed the data from your questionnaires, you will probably need to alter your session according to the results, repeat the session in its amended version and then re-evaluate it. Remember that the process of evaluation and the development and redevelopment of your teaching should be an ongoing process.

HOW TO EVALUATE LEARNING

Much of this topic has been covered in the earlier section on self-evaluation as this relates to all learners, whatever their role or course. Your learners should be encouraged to undertake a process of self-evaluation related to both theory and practice. Many of them will also be encouraged and expected to produce a reflective diary (see Chapter 4). It is almost impossible to evaluate teaching without evaluating what learning has taken place so you can apply all of the topics discussed in the previous section when you evaluate learning. As can be seen from the questionnaire in Box 7.4, the questions evaluate not only teaching, but also learning. For example, question 7 asks the learners about their ability to link theory to practice, which, if answered positively, suggests that the success of the teacher has enabled the link to be made. Likewise, in question 8, a positive answer suggests not only the learning of a skill, which is within the scientific approach to evaluation, but also a level of confidence in the learner that could allow him to undertake the skill in the clinical situation. This question investigates the additional learning, using the illuminative approach to evaluation.

It can thus be seen that many of the topics already covered in this chapter refer to all learners in your clinical environment. However, there are some methods of evaluation that focus primarily on evaluating teaching. Implicit within responses is the notion that it was the teaching strategies used that enabled learning to take place.

Probably the most obvious way for you to evaluate the learning that has taken place is through the assessment of learners in your workplace. Remember that assessment normally takes place before evaluation, but the results of evaluation feed into the next cycle of the planning and implementation of your teaching, which leads to the assessment of the next group of learners, and so on. Chapter 4 covers methods of assessment that you can use with any learners in your practice area. Now you need to collect the information gathered through assessment and feed it into evaluation. Sound evaluation does not simply rely on information from one source but uses as much information as possible from every source, method and process available to you.

ACTIVITY 7.12

Take about 30 minutes and skim through Chapter 4 and this chapter so far, making a list of all issues that will demonstrate success in learning.

Your list might include:

- motivated learners
- a motivated teacher with the appropriate knowledge and skills to teach the topic
- an environment conducive to learning
- clearly defined and achievable learning objectives, which may be set out in a learning contract and agreement
- a sound link between the practice setting and the educational establishment
- support for both learners and teachers/assessors
- the use of appropriate methods of assessment that give the information needed for evaluation
- time!

Evaluation should show up where any problem lies if it is shown that learning has not taken place, and it can, therefore, give you some information on how to improve this for the next time.

Peer evaluation

One area that applies to the evaluation of both teaching and learning is peer evaluation. Within the evaluation of learning, Burnard (1988) suggests that peer evaluation can follow immediately on from the process of self-evaluation by sharing your self-evaluation within a small group and inviting group members to comment and offer feedback. This process has the advantage of developing self-awareness and can be used, perhaps more appropriately, when evaluating a module of learning.

There are disadvantages to this process inasmuch as it can be difficult to confront your own failings, but to have your peers confirm these findings, even constructively, can be both disheartening and destructive (see the section on 'Feedback' in Chapter 4). In order for peer evaluation to be considered worthwhile, it needs to be ascertained that the group involved is cohesive and supportive, with self-confident individuals who are also confident in their peers, and that the group facilitator (which may be you as the teacher) can handle the session well in order to achieve a positive and constructive outcome.

CONCLUSION

It is hoped that this chapter has enabled you to differentiate between the processes of assessment and evaluation, and has, therefore, helped you to use both processes accurately and appropriately.

Nurse educators, including practitioners who teach as part of their role, need to be as actively involved and committed to the whole process of evaluation with their learners as they are to the evaluation of patient/client care. The ultimate aim of any evaluation process is to learn from mistakes, identify and build on examples of good practice and eventually develop the best possible processes for the delivery of the next programme of learning.

The evaluation of teaching and learning can help you to develop a level of autonomy and independence vital within current health services and nurse education systems. You need to ensure that learners, including yourself, accept accountability for and the ownership of learning. The use of learners, peers and yourself in a variety of methods of evaluation will ensure that everyone is involved in developing the best possible systems for teaching and learning.

GLOSSARY

Closed questions: questions that warrant a one-word answer, for example, 'Did you enjoy that session?'

Criterion referenced: a set standard, such as an S/NVQ unit, which is to be achieved during assessment.

Formative assessment: ongoing assessment throughout a learning process.

Illuminative evaluation: the evaluation of the add-on-benefits of learning.

Learning environment: any area, classroom, ward, nursing home, community, etc. in which learning can occur.

Open questions: questions that require a sentence or more to answer. For example, they may ask your opinion on something.

Qualitative data: data related to opinion or information that give some idea of quality.

Quantitative data: data related to numerical scale or analysis that produce measurable facts and figures.

Scientific evaluation: a method of evaluating easily measured facts or items.

Summative assessment: a type of assessment usually used at the end of a period of learning.

Trainee assessor: practitioners undertaking a recognised programme of assessor preparation.

Trainee teachers: practitioners undertaking a recognised programme of teacher preparation.

REFERENCES

Andrew M (1996) Using reflection to develop clinical expertise. *British Journal of Nursing*, 5(8), 508–513.

Burnard P (1988) Self evaluation methods in nurse education. *Nurse Education Today*, 8, 229–233.

Ellington H, Percival F and Race P (1993) *Handbook of Educational Technology*, 3rd edn. London: Kogan Page.

Reece I and Walker S (1997) *Teaching and Learning – a Practical Guide*, 3rd edn.

New College, Durham: Business Education Publishers.

Rogers A (1994) *Teaching Adults*. Milton Keynes: Open University Press.

United Kingdom Central Council for Nursing, Midwifery and Health Visiting (1997) *PREP and You*. London: UKCC.

Ward-Griffin C and Brown B (1992) Evaluation of teaching – a review of the literature. *Journal of Advanced Nursing*, 17, 1408–1414.

FURTHER READING

Cowman S (1996) Student evaluation: a performance indicator of quality in nurse education. *Journal of Advanced Nursing*, **24**, 625–632. *This paper details research that compares Project 2000 students in Northern Ireland with students in the apprenticeship programmes in the Republic of Ireland. The study was derived from the increasing demand for economic models of nurse education as a process within a wider economic agenda. The paper allows readers to extend their knowledge base in this area and to look at issues from a different perspective.*

Reece I and Walker S (1997) *Teaching and Learning – a Practical Guide*, 3rd edn. New College, Durham: Business Education Publishers. *A really useful generic text, which gives the reader some helpful tips in relation to teaching in a variety of contexts. It covers some issues about assessment and evaluation processes that the reader can then apply to the workplace.*

United Kingdom Central Council for Nursing, Midwifery and Health Visiting (1997) *PREP and You*. London: UKCC. *This small and readable booklet explains simply the ramifications of PREP and the processes of which individuals need to be aware.*

Index

Page numbers in bold refer to illustrations and tables